Praise

'When Paul and I started John Paul Mitchell Systems forty-five years ago, we knew that when people feel good about how they look, they are happier and more confident. With this in mind, we created products that enabled people to recreate and maintain their hairstyles at home, between visits to their hairdressers. Leslie Spears and his co-authors have taken this to the next level with *Hair Happiness*, empowering readers with the reasoning and tools to have more effective communication with their stylists, and be more loving towards their hair – which is something that everybody should be able to do!'

— **John Paul DeJoria**, Co-Founder and Chairman, John Paul Mitchell Systems

'Leslie was one of the most inspirational men that I have ever had the privilege to know. To the very end, all Leslie wanted to do was to pass on to others all that he had learned in life. Leslie knew just how important your hair could be. Hair can change your life, be the difference between success, failure and good fortune; and that's what this book can bring to you. Leslie and his co-authors have tackled this subject with sensitivity and skill, drawing upon their combined expertise in business and personal development. This is a thoroughly unique book that will serve as a catalyst to change many lives in the same way that 365 Day Hairdressing did for salon owners and tens of thousands of hairdressers.'

— **Mike Balfour OBE**, Co-Founder, Fitness First

'Even after his passing, Leslie continues to teach us every aspect of hair and haircare. Always the professor, always the businessman, Leslie had the incredible talent to connect the art of hair with the business of hair, and because of that, so many of us have been shown the road to finding our unlimited potential. Personally, I am so thankful I was able to call Leslie my very good friend for many years. I am so pleased that others will be able to tap into Leslie's wisdom and that of his co-authors, Keith, Sharon and Alison, thanks to this book.'
— **Luke Jacobellis**, President and CEO, John Paul Mitchell Systems, retired

'What a joy and privilege it is to see Leslie's wisdom and passion for hairdressing and the success of hairdressers captured so beautifully in this book. His teachings have shaped and inspired decades of my life, and I'm deeply grateful that his generous spirit lives on through these pages – for those of us who knew him well, and for all those who will come to know him through these words.'
— **Debbie Digby**, Founder, Feathers Salon Group; CEO, Passion4hair; NHBF Board Director; Hairdressing Council Committee member

| LESLIE SPEARS | KEITH CHANDLER | SHARON DALE | ALISON COONEY |

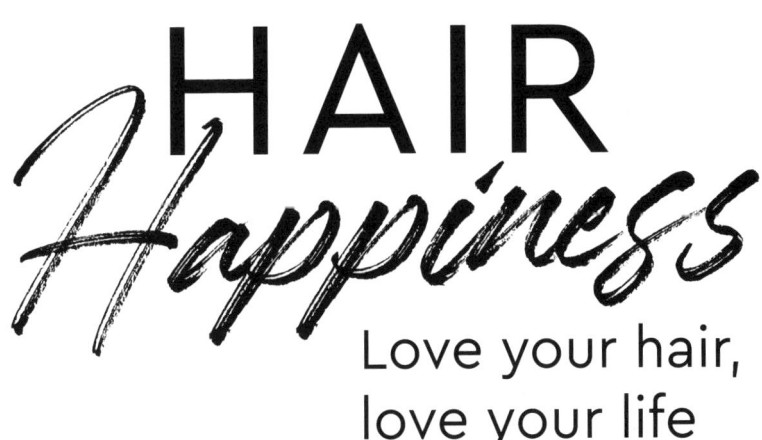

Love your hair,
love your life

Re^think

First published in Great Britain in 2025
by Rethink Press (www.rethinkpress.com)

© Copyright Keith Chandler and George Spears

All rights reserved. No part of this publication may be reproduced, stored in or introduced into a retrieval system, or transmitted, in any form, or by any means (electronic, mechanical, photocopying, recording or otherwise) without the prior written permission of the publisher.

The right of Keith Chandler and George Spears to be identified as the authors of this work has been asserted by them in accordance with the Copyright, Designs and Patents Act 1988.

This book is sold subject to the condition that it shall not, by way of trade or otherwise, be lent, resold, hired out, or otherwise circulated without the publisher's prior consent in any form of binding or cover other than that in which it is published and without a similar condition including this condition being imposed on the subsequent purchaser.

To Leslie, a rare character, a gift to humanity, a beacon of positivity. A brilliant man whose immense intellect and sharp insight transformed an industry and the lives of countless individuals within it. A truly enlightened leader who challenged and inspired so many to unlock their unlimited potential, viewing every interaction as a teachable moment – an opportunity to laugh, learn, achieve, improve and ultimately create joy in the world.

Contents

Foreword		1
Introduction		5
1	**What's Hair Got To Do With It?**	**11**
	You do care, really	11
	The changing face of happiness	12
	Guilty or not?	14
	Look good, feel good	16
	How compliments help change our world	18
	The gown we never take off	21
	How will you know you have achieved hair happiness?	24
	Learning checklist	26
	What's next?	27

2	**Who You Gonna Call?**	**29**
	Purveyors of happiness	29
	A quiet revolution	31
	The changing face of the hair industry	34
	Who does your hair?	36
	Educating yourself and finding the right hairdresser	38
	Learning checklist	40
	What's next?	41
3	**Knowing Me, Knowing You**	**43**
	Comparison is the thief of joy	45
	Talk yourself happy	46
	The unsung hero of our appearance	48
	Why are you having a haircut?	50
	What's influencing your choice of style, salon and hairdresser?	53
	Choosing a haircut	55
	Choosing where you go for a haircut	61
	Learning checklist	64
	What's next?	65
4	**Is Anybody Listening?**	**67**
	Explaining what you want	68
	What exactly is communication?	72

Listening to your hairdresser	76
Take charge of your habits	78
Behind the scenes: Typical clients	80
What if you are not satisfied?	82
Learning checklist	84
What's next?	85

5 Don't Let Me Be Misunderstood — **87**

Teamwork makes the dream work	87
Forming good habits	92
Over to you	100
Learning checklist	103
What's next?	104

6 Get Ready — **105**

What is hair and why do we have it?	106
Know your type of hair	109
Hair health	114
How to repair and work with damaged hair	118
Ageing gracefully	121
Measure twice, cut once	122
Learning checklist	125
What's next?	125

7	**More Than A Pretty Face**	**127**
	Greater than the sum of your parts	128
	Speak up	136
	A picture paints a thousand words – the lookbook	138
	Pre-appointment consultations	140
	More than a snap decision	144
	Learning checklist	146
	What's next?	146
8	**It's Not What You Do, It's The Way That You Do It**	**147**
	The best version of you	147
	Others' judgement of you	149
	Your judgement of others	151
	Why do we make judgements?	153
	How to reserve judgement	154
	Get your morning D-DOSE	156
	Learning checklist	158
	What's next?	159
9	**Keep Talking**	**161**
	The full picture	164
	Learning checklist	168
	What's next?	169

10	**Do It Yourself**	**171**
	Life cycle of a haircut	173
	Product tutorial	175
	Tool tutorial	180
	Colouring your hair	189
	Hair extensions	193
	Bringing it all together	193
	Learning checklist	195
	What's next?	196
11	**Simply The Best**	**197**
	What makes a great hairdresser?	198
	A collaborative approach	209
	Doing something for the greater good	212
	Great value for money	213
	Shift your mindset	213
	Learning checklist	216
	What's next?	216
12	**There's Nowhere Better Than Home – Or Is There?**	**217**
	Deciding where to get your hair cut	217
	Pause for thought…	220
	Do they keep their skills as sharp as their scissors?	221

	Beyond continuing professional development	222
	Social creatures	224
	Perils of too little variety	226
	What can hairdressers do about this?	227
	Learning checklist	228
	What's next?	228
13	**Gut instinct**	**229**
	The second brain	230
	We are what we eat, but all is not lost	232
	Mind–body connection	233
	Make the change from the inside out	234
	Talk to a professional	236
	Learning checklist	236
Conclusion		**239**
Notes		**243**
Acknowledgements		**247**
The Authors		**251**

Foreword

Not long after my partner, Sarah, and I formed our portrait business, one of our clients, who happened to work with Leslie, introduced us. She shrewdly suspected we might get along and he would love my work. Luckily (for me at least), she was right, and we instantly hit it off.

I remember that meeting clearly: we sat chatting over a coffee, laughing and talking poetry, portraits, positivity and the power of the human spirit. I came away buzzing.

That was the joy of the man. Sometimes challenging, always interesting, invariably curious and inciteful, never hostile and always with that characteristic glint in his eye. Yup, that glint still makes me smile when thinking about it – and it was especially apparent when he was talking about family and friends.

Leslie could be serious when he wanted to be (he could be the most probing inquisitor), but I never saw him agitated or frustrated. Those emotions would have been far too restrictive for him. Instead, he would turn the conversation to discuss the positives, always the positives. Looking to the future, never to the past.

That's not to say he couldn't point out flaws in someone's approach (ours included), but it was never in a superior or derogatory way – far from it. Somehow, whenever I left his company, my head would be spinning with ideas for doing things differently. To call Leslie a positive force would be an understatement.

There were so many things I could talk about, but ultimately, it was that glint in his eye and his irrepressible joy at simply being there in that moment, whether having a cup of coffee one-on-one or presenting to an entire room of people, that stood out.

He was a rare character indeed, and I will cherish those memories forever.

This is why the book is so special. Until now, only those who met Leslie personally or were fortunate to work with him or enrol in his training programmes were blessed to experience his brilliance.

Ever benevolent, he long held a vision to broaden his reach so anyone who wished to could benefit from the priceless lessons he learned as he overcame many seemingly insurmountable challenges in his life, demonstrating time and time again that any of us can achieve what we truly believe in.

As an industry immigrant (his term), Leslie viewed the hairdressing industry from a completely fresh perspective. He saw a workforce of highly talented people who had long been undervalued. With characteristic ingenuity, he spotted an opportunity to help hairdressers elevate their worth and the public's perception of their work, going on to disrupt the industry with 365 Day Hairdressing.

Not content with transforming the lives and careers of so many in the hairdressing industry, Leslie committed himself to raising the status of hair in our lives, which he believed would further improve standards in the hairdressing industry and the esteem in which we hold hairdressers. He decided to do so by writing this book.

While heartbreaking circumstances have prevented Leslie from seeing it published, it warms my heart to know that, as a result of this precious book, many more people will benefit from his genius. Although we can no longer be with Leslie in person, he remains with us in spirit through this book.

Paul Wilkinson Hon FBIPP, FSWPP
Paul Wilkinson Photography

Introduction

When I first met Leslie Spears over fifty years ago, little did I realise this synchronistic moment would herald the start of a friendship and newfound love that literally changed my life.

It was 1973, and we were working corporately in the automotive industry; I was in distribution, and Leslie was in vehicle rental. A veritable meeting of minds, it quickly became apparent that we shared many values and had the same business principles and ideologies.

It would take over a decade, but you could argue the stars eventually aligned, bringing us together in a business partnership that flourished for over thirty years, during which we travelled the world practising our love for education in an industry so dear to our hearts – the hair industry.

Throughout a life troubled by chronic illness, Leslie often spoke of his wish to articulate his philosophy and lessons learned in a format equally appealing to hair professionals, their clients and anyone interested in personal grooming. That is why we wrote *Hair Happiness*.

To quote Leslie:

> 'Every day is a gift of opportunity to laugh, learn, improve. To make someone happy and to be happy. We believe in you and what your hair can do for you. We believe in ordinary people doing and achieving special things. We believe in an unlimited you. The journey can start anywhere, but we think your hair is a great place to start. And why not? The role of our hair in our self-esteem and well-being is greater than many might realise. In this book, we will show you how a routine hair appointment can become the start of something amazing, where you become the unlimited you, achieving overall happiness and hair happiness in the process. This book is our gift to you. Enjoy it, learn from it, and then go and book your next haircut and put everything we've shared with you into practice.'

INTRODUCTION

If I asked 'Does your hair please you?', while some of you would say yes, most would probably reply 'It's OK,' or 'It bugs the hell out of me.' You deserve better. By reading this book – and accessing the resources within it – you are well on the way to changing that.

Leslie and I have written this book for you, the person on the street, to give you the insight and tools to allow you to ask more of your hairdresser if you need to. At the same time, we want to shine a light on the invaluable role our hair and, by extension, hairdressing plays in all our lives and happiness, and just what amazing and incredibly talented people hairdressers can be. If you're a hairdresser, we encourage you to read the book as well – we hope our perspective on hair and the hair industry will provide you with plenty of food for thought.

Keeping true to Leslie's spirit, we have endeavoured to create a book that is inclusive and takes into account all age groups, genders, ethnicities, neurodiversity and so on. If there are any places where we haven't hit the mark, please know that the intention was there. On that note, we have used the terms 'male' and 'female' for ease in referring to styles traditionally worn more often by men or women. We recognise, though, that hairstyles are fluid, and these definitions are constantly changing. Furthermore, the terms 'men' and 'women' include anyone who defines themselves as such. Likewise, as has become standard in the hair industry in recent years, we have moved away from classifying hair by ethnicity, instead using physical descriptors of hair types (straight, curly, coily, etc) to reflect that, in reality, the lines between ethnicities are blurred.

Having said that, *Hair Happiness* hasn't been written for everyone. No book can be. This book is not for you if you aren't curious about what life can offer beyond your current experiences. However, if you are looking for new perspectives to help you expand your potential, you are in the right place. As you read, you may find that you already practise much of what we share. If that's the case, don't put the book down – keep reading. Validation is as valuable as learning something new. Besides, we are confident that in these pages you'll find something you haven't tried or considered before.

Years of experience successfully changing the lives of salon owners and hairdressers have made it clear to us just how much of a role hair can play in all of us fulfilling our potential. Maybe that sounds far-fetched, but stick with us, because we aim to convince you by the time you finish this book.

Packed full of practical tips and advice, it will take you on a journey, starting with understanding the role of your hair in your happiness, and taking you step by step through how to enhance or even transform your relationship with your hair and, by association, yourself, as well as with your hairdresser. Importantly, we

INTRODUCTION

want to note that great hairdressing doesn't have to come with a huge price tag. We believe in hairdressers earning their worth, but likewise, we believe in you getting value for money for your haircut. The advice we give you in this book will empower you to do that.

Whether you read it in the order in which it was written or you jump about, whether you find it validating or enlightening, we hope you'll find that this book positively impacts your life and your future – and helps you to achieve your own hair happiness.

Despite failing health and his sad passing in 2024 preventing him from seeing the book through to completion, Leslie's passion for sharing his hard-won knowledge and wisdom is clearly present throughout. We were also privileged to have Sharon Dale and Alison Cooney as co-authors. As top stylists with whom we'd worked for over thirty years, they brought a wealth of professional knowledge and unrivalled hands-on expertise to this project.

Although Leslie did not live to see his book published, his spirit and passion infuse every page and word we've written, bestowing on the reader a gift so quintessentially him – a practical, real-life approach to his relationship with, as he called it, 'the gown you never take off'.

A precious legacy, this book is a tribute and a testament to Leslie's extraordinary contribution to an industry he dearly loved. One to which he devoted over half his life, transforming the lives and careers of countless hairdressers and salon owners and their customers for the better. He will continue to do so through this book.

Keith Chandler

1
What's Hair Got To Do With It?

Why is your hair so important to your happiness? Why all the fuss? It's simple. The role your hair plays in your overall appearance is more influential than you could ever imagine. 'What has my appearance, not to mention my hair, got to do with my happiness?' you ask. 'Surely, we've been told not to judge a book by its cover.'

You do care, really

First things first. What best describes you? Are you someone who takes care of themself and their appearance most days? Or are you the kind of person who doesn't bother much? More to the point:

when was the last time someone complimented you on your appearance? Can you remember?

Hold those thoughts as you read on. Despite valid arguments in recent years that humans are not built to be consistently happy (rather, we are designed to survive and reproduce), we have learned from our decades of experience working with thousands of people from many walks of life that most of us nevertheless have an inherent drive to seek happiness.[1]

Even if you answered 'I don't really care' to the above question, we would argue that, deep down, you do. Whoever you are, this book will help you unlock everything you need to know when pursuing happiness – in which your appearance, including your hair, plays an indisputable role.

Excited? Intrigued? Keep reading. Not convinced? Keep reading because we are confident that by the time we're done, you'll realise the value of your hair in your happiness.

The changing face of happiness

We get one life, and, in our experience, most people will tell you they want a happy one. What makes a happy life will differ for each of us, as will the definition of happiness.

Given the events of recent years, how you regard happiness will have likely changed: the global pandemic and its aftermath have shifted our outlook on life, from increasing conflicts signalling a growing threat to world security and life as we know it right down to the effects of global warming and the cost-of-living crisis.

Happiness has become contingent less on the material and more on who we are and how comfortable we are in our own skins, as well as the people we choose to surround ourselves with, in real life and virtually.

If the past few years have taught us anything, it's that life can change in an instant. Considering this, our mindset and its influence on our happiness will play the biggest role in whether we sink or swim. Smile and the world smiles with you.

With the growing emphasis on happiness coming from within, it has never been more important to understand that your ability to feel happy in yourself is, whether you like it or not, influenced by how the outside world reacts to you, be it one person or tens of thousands of social media followers. It is an inescapable truth, no matter how much you might try to convince yourself otherwise: no one is immune to the behaviours of others.

What's more, it has never been easier to exert your opinion on those willing to listen, including people you have never met or are unlikely to meet. No matter whether it was well received or not, or whether you were the giver or receiver, the extent to which we can share our innermost thoughts with others leaves us vulnerable in a way that has never before existed, and this alone can profoundly affect our happiness.

Guilty or not?

How much does your appearance count? A lot more than you may think. Like it or not, you are judged by how you look. In one study, identical trial papers from a theoretical legal case were circulated to a group of judges for them to share opinions on what sentence the defendant, found guilty, should receive.[2]

Half of the group were given trial papers that included photographs featuring the defendant with well-groomed hair wearing a suit, white shirt, collar and tie. In the trial papers given to the other half, the photographs portrayed the same person wearing a studded leather jacket, with their face, neck and hands covered in tattoos featuring offensive words and symbols.

The judges in the latter group issued sentences of up to a third longer.

If your appearance signals 'I don't care about myself most days', others will begin to agree with you. If you

WHAT'S HAIR GOT TO DO WITH IT?

care so little about yourself, the message it will give off, rightly or wrongly, is that you are likely to care as little about others, too.

If this describes you, perhaps in our ultra-connected world you have found a group of like-minded people who accept you the way you are, but if you are reading this book, we suspect that deep down, you are not happy with the status quo and you want to change. In that case, note this: how much effort you put into your appearance *will* dictate whether it works for or against you.

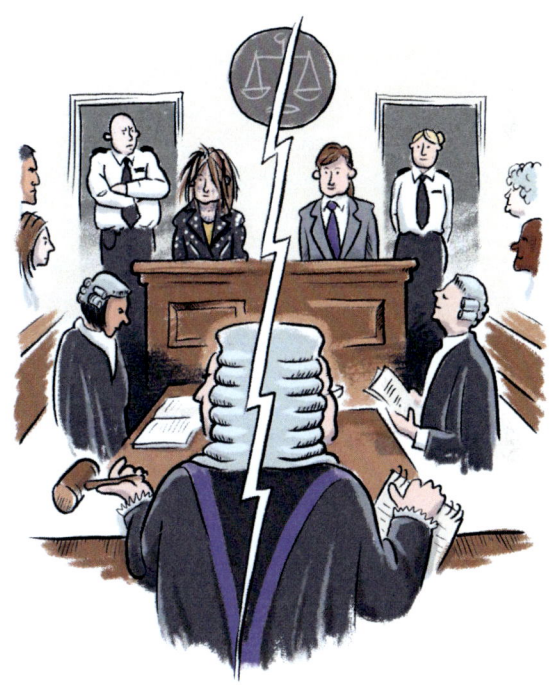

Judged by how you look

Later in the book, we will talk about the role of reserving judgement in your happiness. Still, the fact remains that most people make instantaneous judgements and assumptions, and there are a growing number who will happily share them with the wider world, especially now the wider world is at our fingertips or moments away on a live stream.

It's human nature. Not doing so takes practice, so for most people, it's a habit they won't consider changing, especially if they have a following, large or small, of like-minded people who readily validate everything they say without question. Think about those who have become overnight successes only to suddenly be cancelled, often on the whim of an impulsive judgement passed in the highly volatile court of social media.

We challenge you to become a better person by learning to reserve judgement but, at the same time, accepting that you will continue to be judged by others. The arguments we make about appearance, therefore, still hold and will for a long time to come. Use this wisdom to your advantage.

Look good, feel good

The feedback you receive from others will, in turn, influence how you feel about yourself. To be clear, the opinion of others, of course, doesn't and shouldn't have a monopoly on your happiness. We know this is far easier said than done in an age when we have begun to measure our worth by the number of views, likes, comments or shares we receive, or don't; or the praise we are given; or, sadly, the trolling we're subjected to.

Nevertheless, whether you are given a compliment, are criticised or are simply ignored, you will register it – if not on a conscious level, then certainly on a subconscious one.

It is a rare person whose mood isn't lifted by a genuine compliment, with the resulting boost to self-esteem and confidence positively impacting the rest of their day. As we know all too well, criticism can have an equally powerful but opposite impact – some may argue more so – as can being made to feel invisible or irrelevant.

It can feel unjust, but whether you receive a compliment or criticism in response to how you have behaved or acted can come down to the completely subjective, such as whether the person relates to you, and that can be contingent on how you look, as we demonstrated above.

'Good' is a subjective term. By suggesting you take care of your appearance, we are not saying everyone should hold themselves to the same standards. What does looking good mean to you? Whether your hair is simply brushed and regularly trimmed or professionally blow-dried, you wear make-up or go au naturel, is up to you. What feels authentic and comfortable is important; others will read any attempt to be someone other than yourself in your body language, even if they are not consciously aware they are doing it. No matter whether you shop designer or second-hand, get a manicure or just neatly trim your nails, have your hair regularly styled or simply maintained if the signal you want to give to others is one of 'I am comfortable in my own skin' and 'I care', you will draw the connection you need to drive happiness.

How compliments help change our world

We all love to receive compliments – but why? A genuine compliment is a gift of recognition, reflecting the positive impact you make on the world through the actions you consciously take, whether in terms of your appearance or how you behave. For example, one of our clients, let's call her Helen, received three compliments in the space of a week after using a travel set exactly as the hairdresser had instructed, helping her to keep her hair looking fantastic every day. Helen said, 'I honestly can't remember ever receiving complimentary remarks on my hair. Three in a week.' She felt buoyed by the experience.

If receiving a compliment is a life-enhancing experience, giving one is even more so, to the point it can help change the world.

Yes, you read that right. It is a small action that can make a big difference, much like the 'butterfly effect', and will contribute not only to your happiness but also to that of others. In today's world, that's worth its weight in gold, and the irony is that compliments have never been easier to give.

Still, when we talk about a genuine compliment, we don't mean a 'like' arbitrarily given as we scroll through our feed, or an emoji-laden comment tapped out without much thought. We mean words and actions that come from the heart.

The butterfly effect

The theory of the butterfly effect says that a small action may lead to an outcome greater than itself and that the size of the outcome isn't always proportionate to the original action or even directly related to it.

It was first used in meteorology, after it was suggested that the tiny flaps of a butterfly's wings have the potential to create changes in the atmosphere that could lead to a tornado happening elsewhere.

A small act of kindness by one person *could* have a huge impact on another, so never miss the opportunity to give the gift of a genuine and specific compliment – it costs so little and can mean so much.

HAIR HAPPINESS

If you don't wish to pay compliments in the public world of social media, and there are a multitude of reasons why you might not, give them in person, if you can, or privately by DM, email, video call or phone – whichever way you prefer to communicate.

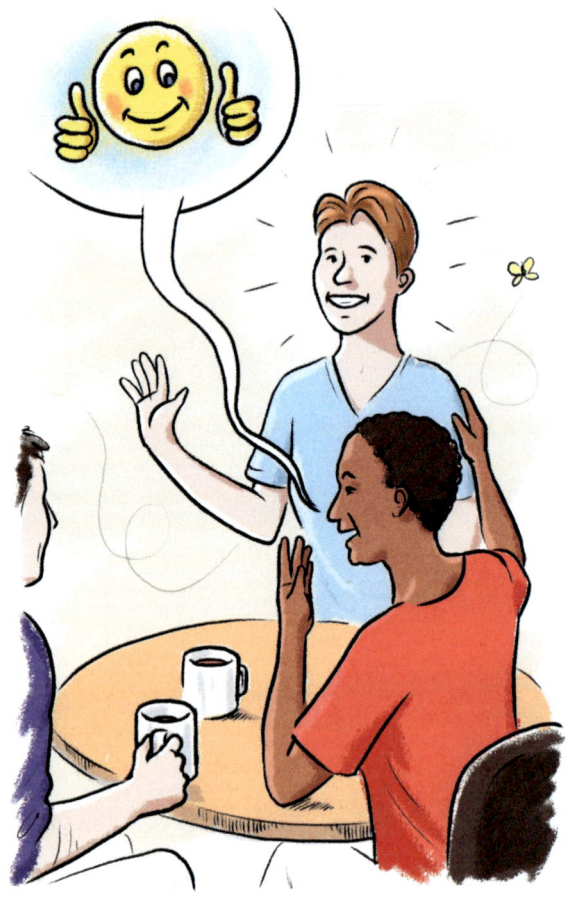

The power of kindness

It is important to know how to leverage the gift of recognition. Never pass up the chance to say 'Thank you, how kind of you to say' or whatever words come most comfortably to you the next time you feel the inner glow of a kind remark. Not only will you be making someone else happy, but you will also increase your happiness.

Look around you. Who are the people who are the happiest? There will, of course, be exceptions, but we will wager that it will be those who are generous with their kindness while clearly taking good care of their appearance. In other words, those who look after themselves and others. They are the ones the world looks most kindly on.

The gown we never take off

Where does hair come in? Millions of years ago, nature gave us hair for physical protection. Today, it helps in different ways. Your eyes are usually the first thing someone notices, whether in person or on-screen, but, as the diagram below shows, how something appears to us is clearly influenced by the size and colour of whatever is placed next to it. Our eyes, face and hair, therefore, are easily enhanced by the magic of well-applied make-up and hair colouring, and our style.

HAIR HAPPINESS

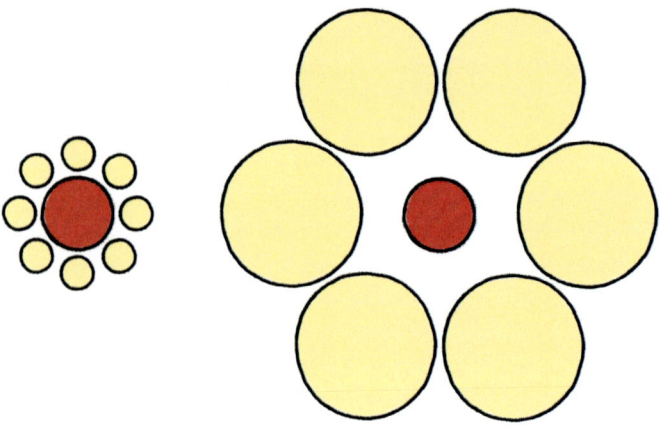

The Ebbinghaus illusion

We have shown these diagrams to thousands of stylists worldwide; typically, over 80% believed the middle circle on the left was larger, an effect named the Ebbinghaus illusion, after its discoverer, the psychologist Herman Ebbinghaus.[3] The rest correctly felt that both circles were of equal size.

As we've established, appearance is paramount and directly impacts our happiness. The role hair plays in how we look is pivotal – it is, after all, the gown or suit we never take off, yet it's given far less credit than it deserves. As you are now aware, our hair's influence lies not only in how it looks but also in how it enhances the shape of our face and even the rest of our body. Whether you are gifted compliments or face criticism or indifference, your hair plays a bigger part than you might imagine.

The power of 365

We set up 365 Day Hairdressing because your hair should work for you and make you happy 365 days a year, not only for the few hours after you step out of the salon, if you want to make the most of your appearance and what it communicates to the world.

One day, not long after he started in the hair industry, Leslie was visiting a salon and couldn't help but notice that many of the clients were heading to the salon restroom directly after having their hair cut. Unconvinced they were all heeding the call of nature, Leslie asked the hairdressers to subtly follow the clients in to see what they were doing. It turned out that, almost without exception, they were rearranging their newly styled hair to something they felt more comfortable with.

Leslie realised the hairdressers were missing a trick: the chance to give the clients a hairstyle they really wanted rather than one the hairdresser felt they should have. It occurred to him that it shouldn't stop there. Clients should be shown how to maintain their new hairstyle between cuts. The idea that would become the 365 Day Hairdressing concept began to take shape, one that holds that a great hairdresser will always put the client front and centre. They will take time to understand what the client wants. They will be curious. They will listen.

A great hairdresser won't just care about your hair on the day of your haircut; they will be concerned about how it will work for you between then and

> your next visit. In addition to the haircut itself, it comes down to the shampoo, conditioner and other products you select, the way you use them and how you style your hair – all things a great hairdresser will show you.

How will you know you have achieved hair happiness?

Only you can answer that question. What we can tell you is that you will have hair that will bring you joy every day. Follow the guidance in this book and you will achieve that. What's extra special is that the happiness it brings will extend to other areas of your life too.

What hair happiness means to Sarah

Sarah achieved hair happiness after a year of hair horror following an allergic reaction to hair dye. Caring for her children and her unwell mother, Sarah had taken to dyeing her hair at home for convenience more than anything.

One day, after a 48-hour patch test had revealed nothing untoward, Sarah applied her usual hair dye. This time, within 10 minutes, it was clear something was not right. Despite her efforts to remove the dye, her scalp became red and sore, and her hair started to smoke.

WHAT'S HAIR GOT TO DO WITH IT?

Diagnosed with chemical burns to her scalp as the result of an allergic reaction, Sarah was told by her doctor not to use hair dye again.

Relieved to still have hair at least, she thought nothing more of it. However, as time went on, her grey roots became more pronounced. Sarah, a confident and bubbly person, began to withdraw into herself. No longer happy with the person she saw in the mirror and shying away from having her photo taken, Sarah felt she had lost part of herself.

To make matters worse, she began to feel bad about how she was feeling. Who was she to get upset about her appearance? Others were far worse off than her. Yet, she couldn't snap out of it, no matter how hard she tried. New outfits, makeup, perfume, not to mention trying hard to believe others when they told her she looked good – none of it worked.

A year on, Sarah felt she had to know once and for all if she could ever dye her hair again. She couldn't go on like this. Searching for local salons, Sarah found Alison (one of the authors of this book). Heading into the pre-appointment consultation, she was full of nerves – afraid of what Alison and others in the salon would think of the state of her hair.

Alison quickly put her at ease, and Sarah said she felt Alison really listened to her as she recounted her story. Rather than judgement, she was met with compassion. 'No one should have to feel like this,' Alison responded, making a commitment to Sarah that she would find a way to help her. Fast forward, and Sarah says not only has her confidence returned, but she is more confident than before. She has fallen in love with herself and her hair again thanks to Alison, who found a way of safely dyeing Sarah's hair again and went above and beyond during that pivotal appointment to ensure Sarah walked away with a stunning hairstyle that she could easily manage.

Beyond that, though, Alison also made sure that after experiencing the trauma of the allergic reaction, Sarah felt at ease throughout the appointment. Confidence in herself, her hair and her hairdresser – that's what hair happiness means to Sarah!

Learning checklist

- Deep down we all care to some degree about how others relate to us.
- This will impact how happy we feel in ourselves. We all seek happiness, even if we have been denying this.
- Our understanding of happiness has changed. It has become more about how we relate to ourselves, the people we choose to surround ourselves with and how we relate to them.
- In today's world, where it is so easy to draw comparisons, judge and be judged, never has it been more important to be happy within ourselves. No one is immune to the behaviour of others.
- We need to take this knowledge and use it to our advantage, staying true to who we are but understanding that how we present ourselves

to the world can have impact – negative and positive.

- Whether we like it or not, appearance plays a role in our happiness – how others relate to us and how that makes us feel inside. Sometimes we won't even be aware of this.
- As the gown or suit we never take off, our hair plays a key role in our appearance. It holds more sway than we may think over our potential to be happy.
- Hair happiness is individual to each of us.

What's next?

Now you understand your hair's pivotal role in your overall happiness – yes, it really is important – we will explore the main players in creating that happiness.

2
Who You Gonna Call?

If your happiness is contingent on your appearance, with your hair playing a leading role, who do you need to help deliver that happiness?

You, of course. Only you can make decisions and take steps to achieve an appearance that results in your happiness, but you will struggle to achieve any of it without your hairdresser. In this chapter we'll look at fixing your hair… and hairdressing.

Purveyors of happiness

As hairdressers, we are responsible for delivering happiness – a truth that has somewhat faded from our collective consciousness. Once a cottage industry, hairdressing has fallen victim to industrialisation. The personal touch has in some quarters fallen away as big impersonal chains have gained a foothold. For some salons, their clients have become commodities and, for the clients, their hair and its role in their lives has been devalued.

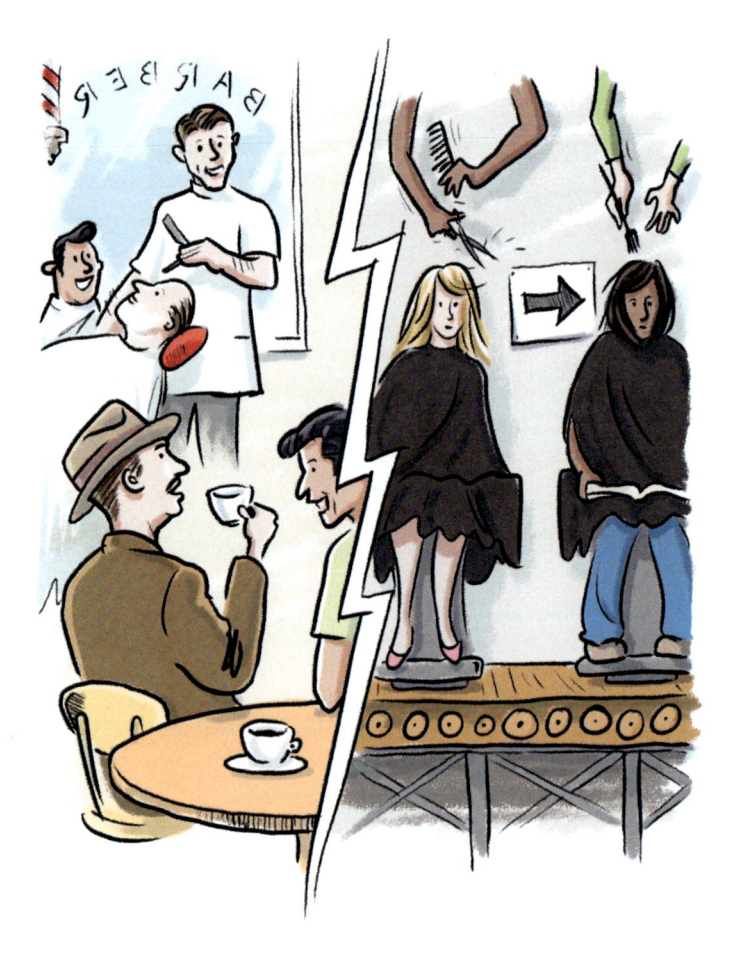

How the salon experience has changed for many over the years

For hairdressing to be seen again as a purveyor of happiness, we, as the hairdressing industry, must bring back the personal touch to all parts of the industry. We can do this in ways that are plentiful, more than at any other time in history, and that our twentieth-century sisters and brothers could only dream about. The tools and technology at our fingertips, which we can use to build bespoke experiences, were unimaginable even a decade ago.

For those hairdressers that have lost it, they need to rediscover the joy and sense of purpose that comes from making a difference in their clients' lives. Salon owners have to find ways of igniting that passion. If you are someone who may have been placing less value on your hair than you should, we, as accomplished hairdressers and industry insiders with a wealth of experience and knowledge between us, can pave the way and show you how to value your hair again and its role in your life and wider happiness. We will show you why you and your hair need to be front and centre of every hairdressing encounter and how, if you accomplish this, you can receive a genuine compliment after every haircut and, more importantly, in between.

A quiet revolution

Crucially, you can help change the status quo by asking this of your hairdresser every time you visit. In other words, share what you know, if it's needed. Help them to raise their own standards. We call it the gift of 'beingness', which means each and every one of us has the potential to become aware of all we are and all we can be, so we can set others up to win, to become their unlimited selves and find happiness, starting with their hair. As Leslie said, 'The only limits to the horizons of your success are your thoughts and actions – then you have no limits.'

Never has this been more valuable than in today's world, where, looking beyond hairdressing, we seem to have lost our way, focusing on our own success and forgetting the value of community and helping one another. We can all play a role in making others' lives better and increase our own happiness as a result. As the adage goes, we can go faster alone but further together.

Change is needed because some of us are placing less value on our hair than ever before, despite its importance. It is often an afterthought in our busy lives. If this resonates with you, perhaps you have been emboldened and lulled into a false sense of security by the wider range of haircare and styling products available online and on the high street. Not to mention the countless styling tutorials that exploded in number during the pandemic. You did it yourself during lockdowns. You can continue to do it yourself now. Because you can 'look after your hair at home', you can go longer between salon visits, you reason. Over time, those visits become further and further apart.

There are others, we know, who have come to value their hairdresser more since the pandemic – you don't realise what you miss until it's gone – yet the increased cost of living means that visits to the hairdresser have become more of an affordable luxury, instead of the habitual expense they once were. Rather than little and often, people are going longer between visits and spending a bit more on each visit. For these people, knowing how to look after their hair between visits has become all the more important.

Where our grandparents and parents would regularly visit the salon – in some cases every week – we're lucky if we manage to squeeze in a visit once every couple of months. Granted, previous generations, particularly the women, took care of their hair to make others happy rather than themselves.

Still, if we can rediscover the joy of looking after and loving our hair for the sake of our self-esteem, self-worth and happiness – or make sure we really know how to look after our hair between visits (especially if we are going less frequently but spending more when we are there), so our hair brings us real happiness between cuts – then we can make a difference in our lives and the lives of others around us because happiness is infectious.

Shortly after making his move from the travel to the hairdressing industry, Leslie was visiting a salon in Ipswich, incidentally one of the oldest towns in Britain. He was shown some salon price lists going years back. He noticed there was no price for a haircut. When he pointed this out to the salon manager, they responded that it wasn't necessary. When people visited salons as frequently as once a week, they wouldn't need a haircut per se. They would ask the hairdresser, 'Please trim this piece for me.' On the next visit, the client would point to a different area and say, 'Please trim this part for me.'

Hairdressing was a frequent purchase and a personal service, with the client making sure they maintained a style that felt right for them. Encouraging regular visits was a practice Leslie adopted in his Mount Street Mayfair salon, where there was a price for a 'Redesign cut', but nobody ever asked for or paid for one.

The changing face of the hair industry

Technology was already changing the industry, but the pandemic, coupled with advances in AI, has only accelerated that change.

Another adage says you never really appreciate something until it's gone. With salons forced to close their doors during lockdowns and find ways to operate remotely, not only did the pandemic highlight how important hairdressers are in our lives, leading hairdressing to be dubbed the fourth emergency service, it also saw a rise in the new kid on the hair industry block: hair coaches, which we will discuss in more detail later.

There has also been an increase in the number of hairdressers opting to become self-employed, facilitated by the opening up of salon suites, giving them a cost-effective, salon-standard space from which to operate. Free from the constraints of long-standing salon rules and regulations, some are leading the way in changing the client–hairdresser relationship by harnessing the power of real-time consultations with existing and prospective clients through direct messaging and chat.

The pandemic also signalled that we need to care more about the environment. Some people have become more conscious about the carbon footprint of regular hair salon visits and the products and treatments they use. This is shaping their decisions around haircuts and styles, with a growing trend towards those involving fewer electric tools.

Coupled with emerging AI in bookings, training and hair consultations, how does this all look for hairdressers? Watch this space. We will briefly explore the impact of AI and related technology on the hairdressing industry in Chapter 6.

Who does your hair?

The answer, 99% of the time, is, 'I do.' In a world where demands on our time come from all quarters, and where we have been led to believe we can take care of our hair equally as well at home and that we're even helping the environment by doing so, making it to a salon is a luxury rather than the regular occurrence it once was. On average, we visit the hairdresser three to five times a year, spending less than twelve hours in total in the hairdresser's chair.

Given the world we currently inhabit, it is unsurprising that we are placing less value on our hair, or have cut down on the frequency of salon visits – although this feels ironic now, we know just how important it is. Along with the ever-growing demands on our time, the growth in chains over the past decades and the associated commoditisation has proved self-perpetuating; if you're getting a factory-style service, you will put less value on your hair and visit the salon less frequently.

Add to that the growing belief that we don't need experts and professionals and that there's a YouTube tutorial or TikTok video for everything. With the cost-of-living crisis, shrinking disposable income will also undoubtedly play a role.

It's down to you to decide if you want to invest your time and resources into more frequent visits to the hairdresser, to continue to put your trust in the professionals who have spent years developing and honing their craft. Nothing can replace regularly putting your hair in the hands of people who make it their business to know and understand what it needs best, by running it through their fingers as well as looking at it. If you are doing all that, then make sure you are asking for the best haircare advice possible from your hairdresser.

Given what we have said about the pivotal role of hair in your appearance and your appearance in your happiness, the issue of time and money, as well as the misplaced sense that you can do it yourself without input from your hairdresser, should no longer be holding you back from giving your hair the love and attention it deserves. If that was the case for you, it may seem more time- and cost-effective to cut down on visits to the salon, but in the end, aren't you just cutting corners?

The frequency should, however, depend on whether your hairdresser has equipped you with the techniques and tools to manage your hair effectively at home – which should come from someone who is acquainted with your hair – so you can go longer between visits should you indeed want to be the one to maintain your hair. Frequency should not be dictated by the amount of time, money and interest you wish to invest in your hair but rather by who you want to maintain your hair – you or someone else – and who is best equipped to do so.

Educating yourself and finding the right hairdresser

What if your hairdresser hasn't educated you on how to manage your hair at home? Then, you would be wise to invest in a hairdresser who equips you with the tools and techniques to maintain your hair expertly between visits – 365 days a year. Again, we are not against teaching you to manage your hair at home. In fact, we were the first to encourage it long before the internet. To attain true hair happiness, however, the advice should come from a professional, not your friend's sister's cousin Liv on TikTok.

Even better, educate your current hairdresser – if you don't want to find a new one. Recommend they read this book. Better them than Liv!

As hairdressers, we must begin to see it as integral to our role to share how to maintain styles effectively between visits with practical styling tips and product recommendations. We know our clients' hair best. Equipping you with the right tools and techniques to make you feel great about your hair every day needs to become second nature to every hairdresser.

WHO YOU GONNA CALL?

We want your hair to look fantastic all the time, not only after you've sat in our chair, so that when you next visit the hairdresser, you do so because the time is right – not because you are overwhelmed or fed up with your hair, or, worse still, because in following Liv's advice, you've done something to it that you shouldn't.

That's not to say you should never watch another of Liv's videos again, but understand that they are there to complement, not replace, your hairdresser. On that note, if you are looking for additional advice that's more professional and tailored than that shared by Liv and friends, a hair coach can work alongside your hairdresser between visits. They are not there to replace your hairdresser, but for hairdressers struggling to find time to support clients between visits, pairing up with a hair coach could be the solution.

A great hairdresser will want you to visit either because you see the value in investing in your hair or because they want you, in partnership with them, to keep it looking, feeling and smelling great 365 days a year. We will share the qualities of a great hairdresser later in this book. We are here to create hair happiness, not relieve hair unhappiness.

As you will now understand, your hair is central to your appearance, which is central to how the world perceives and responds to you. How the world responds to you is inextricably linked to your happiness, whether you want it to be or not, and you have a better chance of the right outcome by first understanding you need a hairdresser in your life and knowing what to expect and, second, investing in a hairdresser that will deliver.

You have an innate need to feel appreciated and supported, which contributes to your happiness and well-being. We all do. Each of us is, moreover, a product of our environment. When you appreciate the importance of your appearance and invest in and welcome a hairdresser into your world who, in turn, invests the effort in helping you look good and feel good both in the chair and between visits, you will feel happier – because a great hairdresser believes in you and your right to feel good about yourself every single day.

Learning checklist

- Great hairdressers should want to be purveyors of happiness – this art has faded somewhat in recent years.

- The challenging times we live in mean many of you are placing less value on your hair – a travesty given what we have shared so far.

- Those of you for whom caring for your hair is still a priority are nevertheless, in most cases, visiting your hairdresser less often.

- If you cannot visit the hairdresser more often, make sure you are asking your hairdresser for the best haircare advice possible.
- You can help change the status quo. You have already started by reading this book.
- To achieve hair happiness, you and your hairdresser need to work as a team.
- You may be lucky and have found the right hairdresser already, whether you see a lot of them in the descriptions in this book or they are willing to develop and take new ideas on board. Or you may need to find a new one so as not to sell yourself short.

What's next?

Now we have established the respective roles of you and your hairdresser and the changes you may need to make, we will explore the common factors that are likely to be driving the decisions you make about your hair, their impact and how to communicate what you want to your hairdresser.

3
Knowing Me, Knowing You

What drives your decisions about your hair and when, where and how often you get your hair cut? We are all unique. We are special. Yet we have characteristics and behaviours that unite us, one being our ego, the driver of our sense of self-worth and self-esteem. Although related to our ego, our decisions about our hair are not self-centred by any measure; rather, they form our intrinsic need to feel good, something we all deserve.

Yes, we're worth it!

What happened when you read the opening paragraph of this chapter? Did you feel a spark of recognition, or did you recoil? Your response will depend on your level of self-esteem, which is a measurement of your self-worth and how much you value yourself. Ideally, you should be comfortable with being unique and, by association, feeling special. If not, we are glad you are reading this book.

The extent to which you value yourself comes into play when you are judged and is effectively managed when you decide to reserve judgement. It is the driving force behind your uplift in mood when you receive a compliment and the opposite if you are criticised or embarrassed or when you negatively compare yourself to others.

Ego

Meaning 'I' in Latin, in simplest terms, the ego is you. It forms your personality, attitudes and beliefs based on your experiences and how you interpret them. It drives how you perceive the world, the choices you make and what happens to you in the future – bad and good.

When allowed to run amok, your ego can give rise to less constructive behaviour. At the same time, it can help you set the boundaries necessary to ensure you don't live your life pleasing everyone else but yourself.

Your ego needs to be effectively managed, of course, by you. It is one of the secrets to living a happy and fulfilled life. After all, it is often said that our most important relationship is the one we have with ourselves.

Your ego is not set in stone. You can change it – one of the premises of this book.

Comparison is the thief of joy

We are all vulnerable to low self-esteem and valuing ourselves less than we should. Engendered by social media comparisons, learning to dislike who we are has become all too easy. The seeds of our discontent can be sown as early as childhood, when we are at the mercy of playground bullies and other negative elements in our lives over which we have little control. Sadly, with the advent of trolling, it doesn't take much for bullying to continue into adulthood these days. It takes nothing to inflict pain on others with a few sharp words fired off from the safe anonymity of a keyboard.

It is easy to forget that the selves we put online are often carefully curated and do not truly reflect who we are – more than likely because of the threat of trolling. We then fall into the trap of wrongly comparing our reality to other people's airbrushed versions of their lives – particularly if we continue to experience the aftershocks of the pandemic, be it a shaken self-esteem and sense of worth or the cost of living. As they say, comparison is the thief of joy.

Despite the perceived negative connotations, your ego and its role in defining your self-worth is both important and necessary, especially in an era of selfies and Instagramming or TikToking, where building someone up and then pulling them down can be done in an instant. Without your ego, you could quickly lose all sense of self-esteem, in which case, you might as well just find a big rock to hide behind. Its existence is why most of us will welcome a positive, 'felt-plus' emotion (a warm, fuzzy feeling) that comes from what for us will be a great hair design and style (beauty will always remain in the eye of the beholder) and why a sincere and genuine compliment always feels so good.

Talk yourself happy

It's not only how others speak to you but how you speak to yourself that counts – your self-talk. It is an integral part of being human and essential to determining how you value yourself.

How you speak to yourself is directly related to your level of self-worth and self-esteem. Typically, 80% of our self-talk is negative, according to conventional wisdom. When we let it run wild, none of it is fact-checked, so we can metaphorically beat ourselves up verbally with impunity.

While we hope you will take joy from knowing that only one version of you will ever exist, accepting and managing the reality of self-talk and understanding its role so it can become more positive than negative will be essential to your happiness.

We need to feel valued, and once you learn how to manage your self-talk – otherwise known as your inner voice or what we at 365 Day Hairdressing called Voice 2 – the opportunities for greater happiness are endless. After all, the simplest way to start is by learning to value yourself. In doing so, you begin to think and talk about yourself in a positive light. Even just the process of thinking and talking about yourself can be the first step in learning to value yourself more.

Thoughts are tools which are only as good as how they are chosen and used for the benefit of your happiness. As Leo Buscaglia, Professor of Education at UCLA, put it in his book *Love*, 'Love does not grow like hair or fingernails; love is a learned experience.'[4]

Before you can hope to achieve hair happiness, you need to learn to love yourself. You need to know and believe you and your hair are worth it. It starts with telling yourself that.

> **Voice 2**
>
> A term we coined for our 365 Day Hairdressing students, we see Voice 2 (otherwise known as your inner voice) as a gift of nature designed to protect us, in the same way as our senses and spatial awareness help protect us from leaning on a hot stove or going too close to the edge of a high ledge. Still, it shouldn't run the show.

> Much like your principal voice – the one you use to speak – you can control what your Voice 2 says to you. We all need some negativity – it can bring clarity and motivate us, stopping us from resting too much on our laurels. If we make the majority of our self-talk positive and empowering, however, we can alter our perspective on life for the better.
>
> For example, your Voice 2, left to its own devices, could be telling you that your hair is simply too unmanageable to bother with. This could result in you neglecting your hair and feeling a sense of dread every time you look in the mirror. Low self-esteem, anyone?
>
> If your hair is 'unmanageable', chances are you've been blessed with unique locks that just need a bit of help to be tamed. Instead, tell yourself that, yes, your hair is spirited, but you've been blessed with something special. Besides, the best things in life take work.

The unsung hero of our appearance

As we have explained, your appearance is connected to your happiness and well-being. You feel good when you look in the mirror and like your reflection – and even more so when others notice and tell you. You might not hear words, but that's your Voice 2 speaking out again, this time on a positive note.

Nature originally gave you hair for physical protection. Now, thousands of years later, hair can help protect you in other ways. Especially in a world where making unhealthy comparisons is all too easy.

If you weren't before, you will now be aware just how much a pivotal role your hair plays in your appearance – the gown or suit you never take off – yet it is often treated as an afterthought despite remaining an integral part of you once you have removed your clothes and make-up.

Considering how easily poor-looking hair can trigger negative feelings – think about all the research supporting the correlation between a bad hair day and a bad mood[5] – not to mention the boost hair that looks and feels great can give you, isn't it ironic that so many of us spend more time on how we choose, wash and care for our clothes and footwear than our hair? We invest far more in a coat, dress, shirt or pair of shoes we wear only occasionally. Is that value for money? Especially in these straitened times?

This is not to say you should forsake other parts of your appearance and focus on your hair alone. Hair is just part of the overall picture – albeit an important one – and a good hairdresser will help you understand how to make it work with your clothes, accessories, make-up and even choice of fragrance in a way that's most effective and gives you the best return on investment.

It's why the hairdressers we trained in our 365 Day Hairdressing system were strongly encouraged to meet and greet every client at reception and to take note of their height, face shape, poise, movement and choice of outfit. We will share tips on this later in the book.

It is also worth remembering that there is more to your hair than meets the eye. We are influenced by all the senses, not just sight, whether judging others or simply satisfying and pleasing our inner self. In this case, touch and, notably, for its ability to trigger a higher recall than any other sense, smell. Nothing beats running your fingers through silky hair – especially when it's yours – or breathing in its intoxicating scent. For this reason, later in the book we will talk you through the importance of using the right products and the role they play in hair happiness (bearing in mind their potential impact on the environment).

Why are you having a haircut?

In the same way that we are connected by our innate need to feel good about ourselves, there are many common traits and behaviours that we have observed in our clients – from what motivates them to get their hair cut to where they go and how often.

Your decision to get your hair cut is influenced by both logic and emotion. While one will drive you to book an appointment, the other will be the reason behind your choice of hairstyle, salon or hairdresser and whether you feel you have satisfied your expectations and achieved hair happiness. As explained earlier, we are more often than not motivated to treat our salon visit as a distress or grudge purchase and book our next appointment so we can relieve our hair's unmanageability and, in turn, our unhappiness. Just to stop it from bugging the hell out of us.

In this context, it is easy to understand why it has become commonplace for people to spend less on their hair than on other aspects of their appearance – which is all the more ironic in times when so many of us need to be more careful with our spending. We are here to help change that. There is significant value in investing in your hair – not least the reward of greater happiness.

After years of observing clients, we have identified the following common reasons that will drive your decision to get your hair cut:

- **Maintenance:** Your hair has become unmanageable; it has grown too long, lost its shape and/or developed split ends. If you dye it, your roots or grey is showing. Other treatments you may have had have started to lose their effectiveness.
- **Event:** You have been invited to a wedding or are getting married. Or you've got a job interview, first date or something similar. You're looking

for a confidence boost and/or want to make an extra-special impression.

- **Life change:** Becoming a parent, going through a breakup or divorce and starting a new job or career are all reasons to refresh or upgrade your appearance, starting with your hair.

- **Time of year:** You may choose shorter hair to stay cooler in the summer months, or decide to go shorter in the winter because of the time it takes to dry longer hair, or opt to use dry shampoo.

- **Habit:** With shorter hairstyles, habits can come into play. You start visiting the hairdresser every two or so weeks to maintain the cut, which is good – or maybe it isn't. Either way, while your decision to cut your hair short was a conscious one (be it for practical purposes, to follow a trend, or wanting a radical change), due to the frequency with which you visit the salon, your behaviour morphs into a subconscious habit, so you may slip into hair unhappiness without realising it. It just becomes something you do. We will go into why we form habits – and how you can use this knowledge to stop bad habits and build good ones – later in the book.

Forming habits aside, what we have shared so far are logical, *rational* reasons. Let's look now at where the emotion comes in.

What's influencing your choice of style, salon and hairdresser?

The deeper, emotional reasons, which, depending on whether they are fulfilled or have satisfied your inner self, will impact how you feel about your hair and your overall happiness. You will doubtless have been familiar with the rational reasons we outlined for getting your hair cut, but have you ever paused to consider what else is driving your decision? Perhaps you recognise some of the following motivators:

- To feel good
- To feel like you belong, for instance, if you like to keep up with trends on social media
- To feel confident
- To feel like you have got a good deal, that you and your custom are valued in that you walk out with a style that captures and brings out the best in you

Your haircut is so much more than what you see on the outside. Yes, you may want to look fantastic for a wedding, a party or a job interview, but deep down, you are seeking a boost in self-esteem and an increase in your overall feeling of self-worth so, for instance, you can move on from the past after a breakup. Your Voice 2 will be whispering, or possibly even shouting, that you need it. Even if you already ooze self-confidence, we can all benefit from a boost from time to time, especially in the challenging world we currently live in.

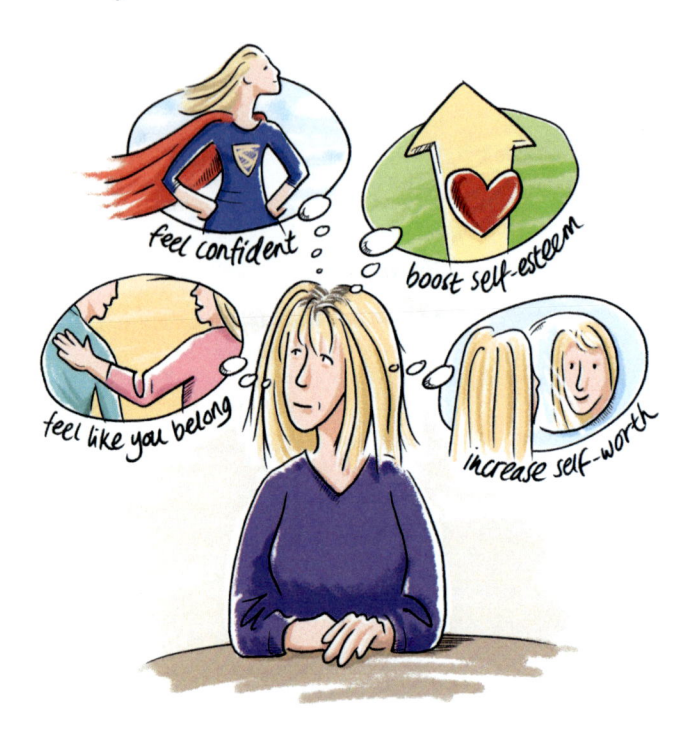

Emotional reasons

This underlying desire to feel confident and like you belong will drive your choice of hairstyle, salon and hairdresser. It will influence whether you are happy with your hairdresser and the outcome of your visit. How did you feel after your last hair appointment? Like you've been tidied up a bit? Ten feet tall with the confidence to conquer the world? Or somewhere in between?

Choosing a haircut

Your deeper emotional reasons will drive your choice of haircut, although it's the rational reasons that will prompt your decision to book an appointment in the first place. In other words, *wants* versus *needs*, although the thought processes aren't isolated.

You will likely build a picture in your mind's eye of the exact cut or style you want, which will be related to why you felt you needed a haircut in the first place, be it a specific or life-changing event. You will perhaps factor in what you know about your hair, including its type and what has worked well for you in the past.

Perhaps you need to boost your self-esteem and confidence. Self-perception and self-knowledge play a role in forming the picture in your head. As we go through this book, we will share how to develop these.

Your health and your hair

Something that has become a more common occurrence over the years is the need for a wig, with cancer and other conditions, such as alopecia, being the main causes. Losing your hair can be devastating, as it is an important part of your identity, and if it comes at a time when finances are tight due to ill health, it can be all the more crushing. Caring and sharing are central to what we did at 365 Day Hairdressing and do now with Joy Ltd, and over the years, we have donated countless wigs to those in need and continue to do so.

Managing hair through cancer treatment

Rachel is a secondary school teacher. When she was diagnosed with cancer, she was reluctant to tell anyone at work and wished to avoid anyone noticing any changes to her hair at all costs. Knowing she would be facing chemotherapy, Rachel didn't want to have to deal with the sympathy of colleagues, no matter how well intentioned, or the insensitive comments about losing her hair that she knew were bound to come from some of the teenagers she taught. She asked Sharon Dale, one of the book's authors and her hairdresser of many years, if she could recommend anything.

Approaching Rachel's situation with compassion and the utmost discretion, Sharon worked with her to come up with ways of cutting and styling her hair to minimise the impact of any thinning showing. Sharon also advised on wigs in the event that Rachel did lose her hair.

In the end, Rachel didn't lose any hair, as she opted to use a cold cap during treatment. Still, the fear was always there. Her cancer treatment left her with disfigurements elsewhere on her body, but they didn't bother her as much as the potential loss of her hair. Her hair was part of her identity, and to lose it would have felt like losing part of herself, even if she could cover up hair loss with a wig.

Knowing Sharon had her back and was there to support her at every step made all the difference.

Caring for your hair while caring for the planet

Something we've only briefly touched on is environmental impact and sustainability. You may already consider the effect of regular salon visits (travelling to and from the salon), the treatments you choose and the products you use (their ingredients and packaging) on the environment. If not, doing so doesn't mean you have to neglect your hair; you can have the best of both worlds. Great hair, guilt-free.

Ask your hairdresser for their recommendations. They may be clued up already, but if not, your asking will signal them that they need to be. A good place to start is finding out what the salon does to reduce its carbon footprint. We will touch again on this in Chapter 6.

Caring for your hair shouldn't mean compromising the planet and vice versa.

How well do you know yourself?

What do you believe you deserve? Do you truly believe you're worth it? What do you believe suits you? Do you think you've got this right? Have you asked for help as we have suggested? All this plays a role in how well your expectations are met – not to mention validating that you and your hair are worth the time and attention.

Do you trust the opinions of others? If not, what's driving this? Are you ready for a change, to put your trust in your hairdresser? You should value self-reliance, as it carries with it the traits of self-discipline and initiative, but so does knowing when to relinquish control to another. Put your happiness in their hands – literally. Let's be clear: not to let them do what they want but what you both decide after a balanced discussion.

Do you feel you can trust your hairdresser based on past experiences? Or is it time to find a new one? If it is, we will show you what to look for in a great hairdresser in Chapter 11.

Following trends

Many of us are driven by the desire to belong and be part of something bigger than ourselves, so following trends can often influence our choice of haircut. As has been the case since the birth of popular culture, few of us haven't wanted at some point to have our hair cut in the style of our favourite sport or music icon (or these days, YouTuber, TikTok or Insta star) – more so now we can follow them on an almost intimate level on social media.

Imitation is the greatest form of flattery, right? Think of Ronaldo's short pompadour. While arguably stylish, this cut is high-maintenance, requiring regular visits to the hairdresser. Is it, therefore, a blessing or a burden?

With longer styles, layers, fringes and framing are in vogue but can be high maintenance, too. Again, is this a source of happiness, which we hope it is – who doesn't like to be pampered by the hairdresser? Or does it leave you short on time and money?

It's worth considering that, while following trends can feed what you *want* in a hairstyle, you should take your work and lifestyle *needs* into account – or fail to do so at your peril.

Jobs, careers and lifestyle

Your job, career and how you spend your time outside of work are also factors in your choice of haircut. This is what we mean when we say your rational and emotional thought processes – your wants versus needs – aren't isolated. How much you let your needs encroach on what you want varies from person to person.

Having said that, the hairstyle needs of a make-up consultant in a beauty store are different from those of a specialist nurse in an operating theatre, a scientist working in a sterile environment or a maintenance worker on a wind turbine miles out to sea, but there will always be evenings and days off when you will desire to look different and feel special.

We will go into more detail about lifestyle and its impact later in the book. For now, understand that it is in your interests to find a balance between what you need daily and what you want when you are free to be completely who you choose to be. There are also factors, such as time and disposable income, suited to maintaining whichever haircut you select. Don't be afraid to raise cost as a reason for choosing a particular hairstyle. A great hairdresser won't judge you for it. If your hairdresser does judge you, it speaks volumes about them as a person and signals that it is time for you to change who cuts and styles your hair.

Returning to the example of someone with short hair and the habit trap, there are three possible scenarios:

- They have the income and lifestyle suited to the haircut and achieve hair happiness.
- They don't have a suitable income or lifestyle but persist, making sacrifices resulting in unhappiness in other parts of their lives.
- They just let their haircut grow out, leaving them disappointed that it didn't work out for them.

This shows why choosing a hairstyle that suits you and your lifestyle is so important.

Are you afraid of jumping out of the frying pan into the fire? Stop settling. Stick with us and follow our advice, and you will be jumping confidently into the limelight. It's your time to shine.

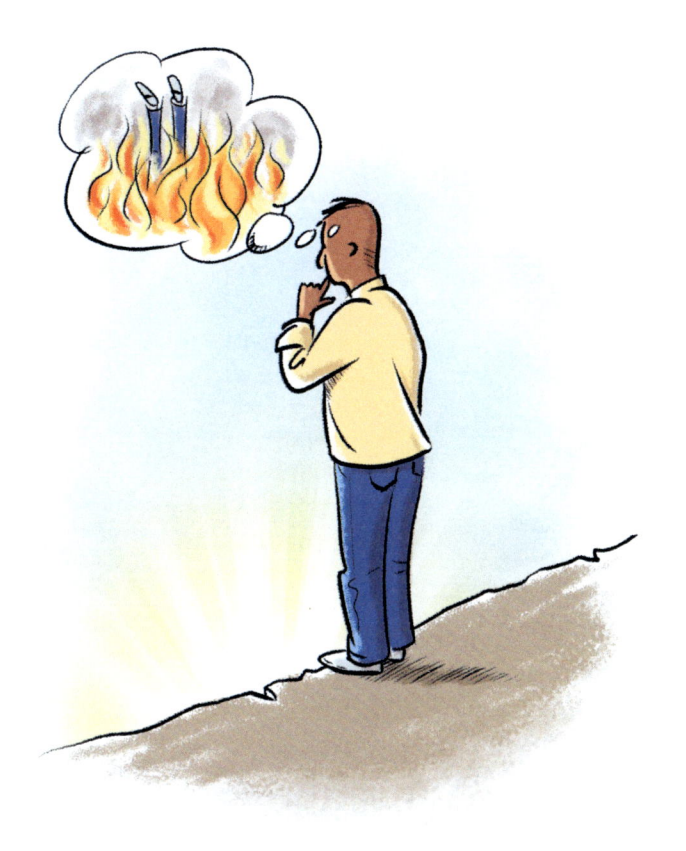

Out of the frying pan into the light

Choosing where you go for a haircut

As you now know, deeper emotional reasons will influence your choice of hair salon or even whether you have your hair cut elsewhere, such as at home or at your hairdresser's home. These decisions are strongly related to how your experiences have made you feel in the past. We will explore the differences between the various options in Chapter 12.

You will also be influenced by financial considerations, as we have touched on above, as well as convenience and, of course, habit.

Loyalty or variety

Do you choose a new hairdresser each time, or a hairdresser who feels like a friend or even part of the family?

As explained earlier, hairdressing services have changed dramatically since the mid-twentieth century. In years gone by, there would have been a salon just down the street that you'd visit weekly to have your hair styled and set. The hairdressers knew you and your family knew them. Because everyone visited the local hairdresser so frequently, they needed only 120 clients to earn a living; it was a truly personal service.

Today, a typical hairdresser in a city salon needs over 350 clients and may therefore fail to remember your name or what you do and won't bother to look it up. They will also continuously need 25% of new clients to replace people who have moved away or opted not to come back after a first visit.

Hairdressers, like all skilled people, have their strengths and weaknesses. Their strengths are likely to blow you away, but their weaknesses can let you – and them – down, especially if they include an inability to understand you and your hair needs. This is often the difference between a well-managed salon and one perpetually needing an additional, above-average hairdresser to commercially survive.

What's driving your preference? Do you want to change, or should you change? If you prefer having a different hairdresser each time, it shouldn't matter which one you team up with if you choose a great salon, if that's your preference. The hairdressers will themselves be a team working to give you the top-notch service you deserve, even when they're having a bad or overly busy day – we all have them.

Teamwork isn't valuable only in work, school or the sports arena – it has value in all areas of life. Every time we put our trust in someone to help us reach for what we want, we are investing in the power of teamwork. It takes time, effort and courage.

Find a hairdresser or hairdressers you can work with, then work with them. Together, you can go far, contributing to one another's happiness along the way. We will guide you on how to select a great hairdresser in Chapter 11.

Frequency

The average person loses about eighty to a hundred hairs a day. While some hairs are growing, others rest or they are shed. It's one of nature's paradoxes: what's dead but still grows? Your hair. Like your nails, but where damage to your nails is noticeable and gets dealt with quickly, the damage to your hair sometimes goes untreated.

If left too long, damaged hair becomes too hard to repair. Your hair, the gown or suit you never take off, needs regular care if it is to continually help you shine. This should be a factor when choosing your next hairdresser or salon.

Learning checklist

- Our hair, as we have established, plays a key role in how we feel about ourselves and how we are perceived by others – they are not mutually exclusive.

- At the heart of how we see ourselves is our ego, which drives our sense of worth and self-esteem.

- Our sense of worth and self-esteem are impacted by how we talk to ourselves.

- How we talk to ourselves can be influenced by what we see in the mirror.

- Our appearance can influence our reasons for going to the hairdresser, which will be both rational and emotional, our choice of hairdresser (whether we've settled for less than the best in the past), where we go, how often and our choice of haircut, or the haircut we agree to.

- Making more informed decisions about the hairdresser you choose will help you achieve hair happiness.

- Your hairdresser is there to help you, which is why it's important you work as a team or find a hairdresser with whom you can work as a team (whether you use the same or different hairdressers each time). Remember, learning is two-way and if there's something you've learned from this book that you think your hairdresser will benefit from, share it with them. It's a gift.

What's next?

Now we've covered what drives your decision-making when it comes to when, why, where and how often you have your hair cut and/or styled, the impact on your happiness and what you can do to mitigate and leverage it, we will explore how to make the most of your time and money in your hairdresser's chair, starting with the need for vital two-way communication.

4
Is Anybody Listening?

A good haircut equals more than good technique. In this chapter, we begin to take you through how to get the most from your visit to the hairdresser and beyond, starting with communication, as great hair results from so much more than the hairdresser's technical skills – although it goes without saying, they are essential. Drawing on what we have observed working with a wide variety of clients over many years, this will lay the groundwork for what's to come as we guide you towards hair that makes you happy 365 days a year.

It's more than talk. When you arrive at the salon or your hairdresser's home, you may not realise it, but you are communicating the moment you step through the door, even though you may not have spoken a single word. Do you walk in with purpose? Or do you shuffle in, embarrassed by the state of your hair? In other words, are you brimming with confidence or are you looking to hide behind the big rock we mentioned earlier?

Think about the messages your body language gives off. Be honest with yourself. Which message is more likely to result in hair happiness? If your body language needs work, we go into more detail in Chapter 8.

Explaining what you want

Once you are sat in the hairdresser's chair, whether as part of a pre-appointment consultation or for the appointment itself, how well do you communicate what you want? Think back to your most recent visit. Did you have a clear picture in your mind that you shared concisely and confidently with your hairdresser, or did you quietly mumble something along the lines of 'a quick trim and tidy'? Were you willing to listen to the recommendations your hairdresser made, or were you so set on what you wanted that you instructed them to do exactly as you asked? Were you at the other end of the scale, waving their questions aside with a 'Do what you like'?

As you might have guessed, when it comes to determining what you want, you will find yourself somewhere on a spectrum. At one end are those who struggle to put any trust in their hairdresser, preferring to come armed with a set idea of what they want from a hairstyle and refusing to entertain any advice. At the other are those who acquiesce without hesitation. Everyone else falls somewhere in between. Ideally, you want to be right in the middle, where you have found a happy medium.

Why? Because if you recognise yourself as being on either end of the spectrum, chances are you won't be communicating with your hairdresser as well as you could, the inevitable outcome of which will be hair unhappiness.

Remember, you are and should be a team.

Those who acquiesce

Over many years of developing and running training workshops on communication for hairdressers, we devised a compelling way of showing exactly what can go wrong when the hairdresser and client fail to communicate with one another.

In front of a room of 500 or more hairdressers, we bring a professional model onto the stage wearing a stunning gown by a leading designer. We tell her we have lined up one of Britain's finest hairdressers to do her hair. The model is shown the hairdresser's impressive portfolio of rich and famous clientele stretching from London to New York.

'Will it be OK with you for him to do whatever he chooses for you?' we ask.

'Yes, of course,' the model replies.

Known as Britain's Finest Hair Ambassador, the hairdresser makes his grand entrance. Circling the model, he examines her hair, gently lifting various sections, feeling the texture and weight and evaluating its shine and depth of colour, and watching closely as he lets go and it falls back into place. He then picks up his portfolio and steps to the front of the stage. With his back to the model, so only the audience can see, he shows the audience his top three choices of hairstyle in order of preference.

The show compère, one of the four authors of this book, then takes the portfolio from the hairdresser and hands it to the model, instructing her to pick her first choice of hairstyle plus two styles she dislikes and doesn't want. A cameraperson using a handheld camera with a live feed running to a giant screen at the back of the stage zooms in on her first choice. It is not one of the hairdresser's chosen three. The room falls into a stunned silence. You can hear a pin drop.

The model is then asked to point to the styles she dislikes, which, as you may have already guessed, are two of the hairdresser's top three. The moral of the demonstration: however good, great or famous the hairdresser, *never*, *ever* say 'Do what you like.'

Choosing a hairstyle must involve two-way communication between the hairdresser and the client. There will be reasons why the hairdresser in the story above made their selection, related to factors such as hair type, face shape and body shape, which we will go through with you in more detail later in this book. There will equally be reasons why the model disliked two of the styles chosen by the hairdresser.

On the one hand, without a proper consultation, there would be little opportunity for the hairdresser to explain his reasons for selecting his chosen styles and for the model to explain why she doesn't like them. On the other hand, were they to speak to one another, the resulting mutual understanding could lead to the model deciding that she does, after all, want one of the hairdresser's top three. Now she understands how it will flatter her face shape, body shape and other features, she likes it.

For those at the other end of the scale, learn to put some trust in your hairdresser. Suggest the style you want but ask for their input. If you don't like what they recommend, ask what's behind their suggestion. Between you, you will come up with a style that will result in hair happiness. With ongoing developments in AI, your hairdresser may even be able to show you what the style should look like on you. A hairdresser who is clear on what you want and don't want and why is less likely to go 'off-piste' when cutting your hair.

Ultimately, you want to reach a point where you have settled on the hairdresser creating a style that they believe best suits you, your lifestyle, hair type, personality and so on, and that is one you are happy and comfortable with, as well as being clear on why it suits you. You can achieve this only with effective communication, and communicating effectively is easier than you think.

How you communicate will also depend on whether you have a long-standing relationship with one hairdresser or prefer switching hairdressers with every visit. Is your hairdresser like family or a relative stranger? There is no right or wrong way, but the approach you take should differ accordingly. The former will know your hair well, to the point you will need to be clear if you want to do something different – like anyone, hairdressers can fall into habits without realising it. With the latter, you will need to be prepared to provide a brief history to your hair each time. We will talk about creating a 'hair backstory' later in the book.

No matter what relationship you choose to have with your hairdresser or the process they follow, achieving the outcome you want boils down to one thing: how well you communicate with one another.

What exactly is communication?

As you've guessed, communication isn't just what you say – it's how you listen, your body language and how you read the body language of others. It

IS ANYBODY LISTENING?

even comes down to mindset and how well you strike a balance between knowing what you want and being open-minded enough to take advice from your hairdresser.

When training hairdressers through our 365 Day Hairdressing programme, we ran a number of exercises that reinforced the understanding that less than 10% (typically 7%) of communication comes from the words we use.[6] With this in mind, how good are you at communicating? Now think about your current or last hairdresser. How would you rate their communication skills?

Are you explaining what you want and, just as importantly, what you don't want? Is your hairdresser listening and taking it in? How can you tell? Can you see it in their body language? Are you listening to them? Are you asking questions to make sure you've understood them? Are you taking their advice and recommendations on board?

Hairdressers will rightly argue that a bad haircut is more often than not down to poor communication rather than poor technique. Think about bad haircuts you may have had. Be honest with yourself – how much did poor communication play a role in these situations? There are some examples of what can support and what can hinder communication in the table below.

Supports communication	Barrier to communication
You listen attentively.	You don't pay attention or you struggle to do so.
You focus on the present.	You focus on what has gone before. You use universal statements such as 'this always happens'.
You ask questions. You never make assumptions.	You often assume you know what the other person means. You rarely ask questions to gain increased understanding.
You hear people out.	You interrupt or struggle not to.
You are willing to compromise and consider an alternative viewpoint.	You are often unwilling to consider a compromise, or compromising and seeing an alternative viewpoint is something you struggle with.
You clearly state what you want or intend and why you believe it matters.	You lack confidence in stating what you want or intend; you agree to whatever is suggested to avoid any awkwardness; or when you make suggestions, you seek permission from the other person using phrases like 'Would you mind if I asked for this…' offering an opportunity for the other person to refuse without learning more about what you want or intend.
You never assume the other person knows what you want.	You often think people should know what you want, or struggle with the idea that people don't always know what you want.
You use words and phrases that the other person can easily understand.	You speak in jargon or use lots of technical phrases.

IS ANYBODY LISTENING?

Although a discussion on neurodiversity and how it can influence communication falls outside the scope of this book, we want to take this opportunity to recognise that neurodiversity can impact communication. If you are neurodivergent and feel comfortable sharing it with your hairdresser, we recommend that you do. Likewise, we recommend neurodivergent hairdressers share their neurodiversity with their clients. Openness, if you are comfortable with it, only aids communication.

Yes, you can walk into the salon (or wherever you choose to have your hair cut) having clearly prepared what it is you want done with your hair, but that is only half the job. Communication is two-way. While you are the expert on *you*, and it goes without saying that any hairdresser worth their salt will take the time to listen to you and ask questions to make sure they completely understand your wishes, your hairdresser is the expert on *hair*. Fail to listen to what they have to say at your peril. At the same time, take heed of the story above, and don't put your choice of hairstyle entirely in their hands.

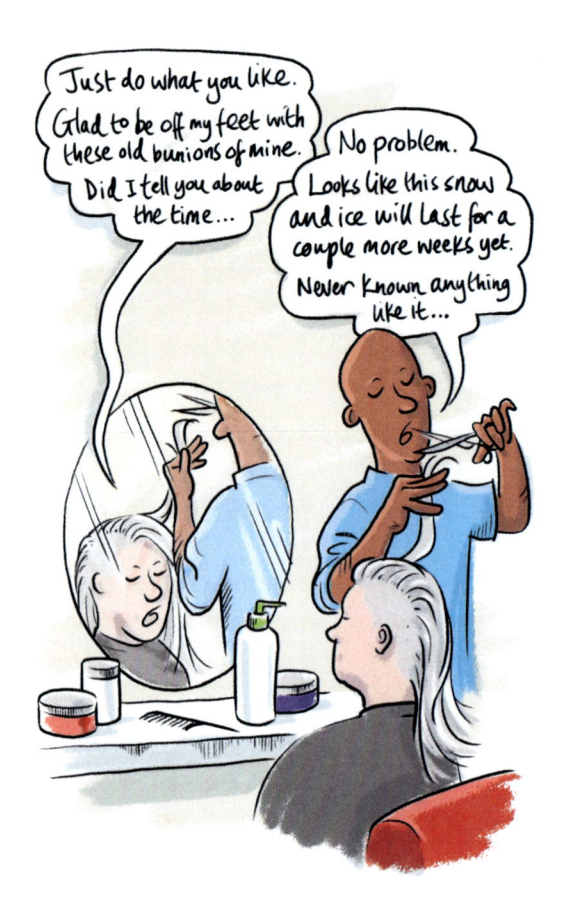

Talking but not listening

Listening to your hairdresser

Are you an active listener? Are you completely present when you are in the hairdresser's chair? Do you listen attentively when they are talking about your hairstyle and giving their recommendations, or do you let your mind wander? Are you busy scrolling through

TikTok, Instagram or messages on your phone? Do you use your time in the chair to multitask and catch up on other things while you let the hairdresser get on with their stuff? If so, *stop*. (Again, if you are neurodivergent, we appreciate this won't simply be a case of telling yourself to stop. We recommend letting your hairdresser know and working with them to determine how you can achieve what we are aiming for here.)

You are not just paying them to cut your hair – you are paying them to give you a hairstyle and, hopefully, the tools to keep it looking fantastic 365 days a year. Listen attentively and be open to their advice and recommendations. Make sure you understand. Reflect. Ask questions if you aren't clear about what they are suggesting or if they are not forthcoming. Be curious. Some things require at least two people to accomplish them well, and this includes hairdressing. We can't emphasise enough, you are a team.

How good are you at taking your hairdresser's advice on board? How open-minded are you? As we've seen, handing over all control to the hairdresser can be perilous, but doing the exact opposite will just as likely lead to hair unhappiness. How easily do you relinquish control and trust others? If the answer is 'not well', what can you do about it? You can't have good communication without trust.

Learning to trust is important. If you answered 'not well', what stopped you trusting? You weren't born that way. How do you learn to trust again? As we have said before, self-reliance isn't a bad quality, but in excess, it can become harmful, especially if you lose the will to trust and forget how joyful it can feel to depend on others and have them depend on you.

It can take courage to relinquish control, but the rewards of a new perspective can be limitless. The right hairdresser will see strengths in you that you didn't know you had and use their skill to leverage those strengths. Life can be lived to its fullest only if we accept the symbiosis of mutually beneficial relationships. The client–hairdresser is one such relationship. Learn from one another.

If the opposite is the problem and you sit on the other end of the spectrum, what led you to put your hairstyle completely in your hairdresser's hands? A run of luck doing just that? It is tempting to always take the path of least resistance – life seems so much easier that way – but in the end, your luck will run out. Remember, your hair deserves more.

Take charge of your habits

Whether it's learning to actively listen, be present, be less passive or trust, the starting point is understanding what stopped you from doing these things in the first place. Meditation and introspection are powerful tools in determining what drives our behaviour and beliefs, as we will touch on in the next chapter. Be mindful and take charge of your habits.

Once we know what formed a bad habit, how do we turn it into a habit we want? We start by understanding why we form habits. Essentially, we do it to save our brain energy. Conscious thought takes energy, which is why any new behaviour takes effort. Once a behaviour becomes a habit, it slips into our subconscious, where we act on it without thinking, saving us energy. Great, if a habit is a good one. Not so great if it's a bad one.

How do you change a habit? You become the director of your own mental movie. Imagine what you'll feel like when you decide to trust your hairdresser and let them create a look for you that blows you away, or you choose to take a less passive role. Then, each day, mindfully recall that feeling so that when you next sit in front of your hairdresser, you have the courage to do it for real.

You won't regret it, because there is more to your hairdresser than meets the eye, including their ability to process information physically through movement and touch, known as body-kinaesthetic intelligence, or through what they observe you doing, known as spatial-visual intelligence. If you ask most hairdressers, however, they are unlikely to have heard of these terms. Why would they? These are things they do subconsciously as a result of natural talent and years spent honing their craft.

You could even go as far as saying this enhanced ability to communicate nonverbally is their superpower. Add to it interpersonal intelligence, through which they can tune into and gauge your mood and emotional state and adapt their approach accordingly, and the sum total is their ability to interpret a whole range of nonverbal signals that you might be giving off. Be it your facial expressions, your movements or your tone of voice, a great hairdresser will be able to determine whether you are nervous and not sure what you want or confident and full of purpose, whether you are likely to want to be involved in decisions about your hair or will try to take a back seat, or whether you are a good listener and are willing to trust or they need to work to gain that trust. Impressive, right?

How about you? What can you tell from your hairdresser by their nonverbal communication? How can you use this insight to achieve the best outcome from your visit?

Behind the scenes: Typical clients

Over the years, we have identified four main types of client based on common attitudes and behaviours, which we have listed in the table below. Alongside each one, we have suggested points that you and your hairdresser might want to consider so you achieve the best outcome from your visit. As you can see, it all comes down to communication.

	Attitude/Behaviour	Considerations for hairdresser	Considerations for you
Client 1	You will be so pleased to be (finally) getting your hair cut.	The client will be happy whatever the outcome but the hairdresser should be mindful not to give in to temptation and cut corners. They should take pride in every haircut they do.	It's great you are so chilled, but remember, you are worth it. Take some time to plan what you want and discuss it with the hairdresser. Don't just take what comes.
Client 2	You see a visit to the salon as an opportunity for special pampering.	The client may well expect more than average. The hairdresser should set boundaries and clearly explain at the beginning what comes as part of the service and what doesn't.	Yes, you are worth it, and it's great that you hold the hair salon in such high esteem, but make sure your expectations are aligned to avoid awkwardness and disappointment.
Client 3	You are looking for a complete change – perhaps you are a divorcee or in midlife/ageing.	The decision for a complete change will be driven by emotion. The hairdresser should, therefore, take time to fully consult with the client before restyling their hair. Otherwise, they risk them hating it the next day.	A complete restyle might seem like a great solution – and it could well be exactly what you need – but take time to pause and consider if it is what you really want. Talk to your hairdresser. Ask them what they think. There may be a middle ground they can suggest.
Client 4	You are anxious and nervous.	The hairdresser should be empathetic. There are various reasons why some people find visiting the hairdresser nerve-wracking. Social anxiety can be debilitating, so they should be gentle and ask what they can do to help.	Know that it is OK. If you find visiting the hairdresser a cause of anxiety, perhaps take a friend with you who can help with talking to the hairdresser and make the experience less nerve-wracking. Also, let the salon know so they can make adjustments to help your visit go as comfortably as possible.

Which can you identify with? You might have been a different type on varying occasions or a combination of types. In addition to our suggestions, think about what you can do differently at your next visit. Again, it essentially comes down to better communication.

Poor communication can result in mismanaged expectations, which will influence your experience and the outcome of your visit. This, in turn, will of course impact your level of happiness with your hair. We will go into typical expectations and misconceptions in the next chapter and how to manage the former and avoid or overcome the latter.

What if you are not satisfied?

If you and your hairdresser have communicated effectively, you will understand the process doesn't finish when you stand up from the chair. How do you feel immediately afterwards? Several days later? Right before your next cut?

If it didn't turn out as expected, how do you turn the disappointment into something positive? If you are not satisfied, learn from it. What could you do differently next time to ensure a better outcome? Be mindful, however, that turning a negative into a positive rests on your ability to refrain from dwelling on what the hairdresser did or didn't do or beating yourself up about what you might or might not have done, if you are that way inclined.

Instead, focus your energy on clarifying what you want and the steps you need to take to turn your haircut into the one you'd hoped for. We can guarantee communication will be in there somewhere. Both you and the hairdresser will learn and grow from the experience because it will be framed in the constructive approach of focusing on what needs to be done rather than the destructive process of apportioning blame.

Your trip to the salon is so much more than a haircut. It's a chance for you to develop the qualities illustrated below – to learn more about yourself and your hair and, in doing so, grow personally as you build self-esteem and confidence or compassion and humility. It is the opportunity to improve how you make the most of your hair between visits and share what you've learned with friends and loved ones, as well as pass it on to hairdressers whose services you use in the future – a great hairdresser will always be willing to learn from their clients. You'll achieve hair happiness and inspire others to do so too.

Let go of the limiting beliefs that have prevented you from becoming the unlimited you!

Philosophy of the unlimited you

LEARN → GROW → ACHIEVE → INSPIRE → SHARE

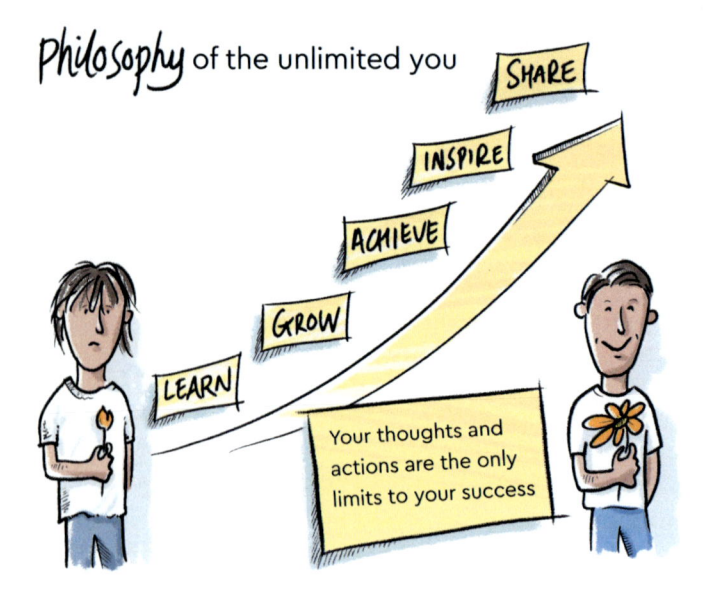

Your thoughts and actions are the only limits to your success

Learn, grow, achieve, improve and share

Learning checklist

- A great haircut is as much the result of great communication as technique.

- Great communication is vital if you and your hairdresser are to work effectively as a team.

- It is important neither to dictate nor to acquiesce.

- Learning to communicate well is a habit that needs to be formed.

- Once you have formed the habit, it will ensure you get the best out of your hairdressing experience, while in the chair and once you have left the salon.

- If you're not getting the best out of your hairdressing experience, and you're someone who likes to stick with a hairdresser rather than have a new one each time, move on or use your newly enhanced communication skills to improve things with your existing hairdresser.

- Use the experience to let go of unlimited beliefs and achieve hair happiness by becoming the unlimited you.

What's next?

Now you are a communication pro, we'll delve deeper into what we have learned clients frequently expect from the wealth of insight we have gathered over decades of working in salons. We will explore what is typically considered a reasonable expectation, what is less so and how and why common misconceptions come about. We will also look at how you can manage your expectations to avoid disappointment, moving ever closer to achieving hair happiness and happiness overall.

5
Don't Let Me Be Misunderstood

It is all well and good becoming proficient in how to communicate, but it means little if you are not starting with the right expectations. In this chapter, we will explore what we consider fair expectations based on our knowledge and experience from years of working in salons across the globe. We will also share common misconceptions and how to avoid them.

Teamwork makes the dream work

You have the right to expect a high-quality haircut and be given the time and attention to ask for advice and communicate whatever's on your mind. You also have the right to a style you can easily manage and guidance on how to manage it so you feel fantastic between visits.

The success of your visit to the hairdresser, however – and, ultimately, hair happiness – depends on you, too: how clearly you share what you like and dislike about your current hairstyle and what it is you might want.

Expectation 1: A technically sound haircut

Expecting your hair to be cut well is, of course, entirely reasonable. You wouldn't walk into a restaurant expecting a poorly cooked dinner or ever expect to stay in a poorly cleaned and maintained hotel room. In fact, you shouldn't settle for anything less than well-cut hair, and if you have done this in the past, we are glad you are reading this book.

The reality is that most of you demand exceptional products and incredible service – and so you should. It hasn't happened by chance. The internet has given you greater access to information than at any time in history, and this will have empowered you as individuals.

Freed from ignorance by the democratisation of information over the last couple of decades, you have grown to expect the best value for money, great products, a first-class service experience and to feel good about yourself and your buying decisions.

As hairdressers, we must embrace this change. If we want you to become an advocate and recommend us to your family and friends, we know we have to deliver a first-class service. It benefits everyone. It encourages us to raise our standards and improve, and, as a consequence, you are rewarded with a better quality of service.

We know that a well-run salon will ensure it delivers the high-quality service you deserve every time you visit, inspiring its hairdressers through its leadership to continually learn and use their learning to achieve, inspire and teach.

Hairdressers who aspire to become the best possible version of themselves will want that for you, too.

We will explore what makes a great hairdresser and salon in Chapter 11.

Expectation 2: Our undivided attention

With the expectation of first-class service, it doesn't come as a surprise that more of you are asking for nothing less than our undivided attention while you are in the chair. You want to feel special and valued. You want your needs met, whether it's us taking our time over your haircut or, if you are time-poor, doing it as quickly and efficiently as possible.

There will, however, be occasions, if we are salon based, when a team member asks us a question or we have to go and briefly help a more junior member of staff. As much as we might want to, giving you 100% attention 100% of the time is not always possible, nor is it needed to achieve a great haircut, although we agree that there are occasions when hairdressers may not give you the attention you deserve. For instance, having your hairdresser gossiping with their colleague while you are fighting to get their attention is not on.

Expectation 3: To look and feel good at the end of your haircut

This is more than reasonable. In fact, we want you to expect more. We want you to look and feel good 365 days of the year – not only when you walk out of the salon (or your hairdresser leaves your house) and for a few hours afterwards but also between visits. We want you to expect your hairdresser to show you how to manage your hair at home – how to style it day-to-day and on special occasions. We want them to guide you on which products and tools to use and how to use them. We will go into this in more detail later in the book.

Expectation 4: That we know intuitively what you need

Who wouldn't want to be a mind reader? Yes, we spoke in the previous chapter about hairdressers having kinaesthetic, visual-spatial and interpersonal intelligence as superpowers, but these powers don't stretch to mindreading. It all comes back to communication. Even if we know you well, we can't know 100% what you want. As we've said, hairdressing is a team effort, which is why a great hairdresser will always be curious and ask lots of questions. We're not being nosy!

Hairdressing is an ever-evolving field. We are constantly learning. If you have come across something new, don't be shy. Share it. A great hairdresser is open to learning and will be willing to listen and hear about anything new you have come across, so never assume we know everything there is to know about hairdressing. You might teach us something.

Expectation 5: That the client is always right

A well-run salon and its hairdressers will always respect their clients. They will never forget that the clients pay their wages and all the other bills. At the same time, they will believe in fairness and honesty. In *what* is right, not *who* is right.

No, the client isn't always right – but neither is the hairdresser or the salon. In fact, no one is right. When it comes to solving issues or settling disputes, a good hairdresser will focus on understanding *what* is the right thing to do rather than trying to ascertain *who* was in the right or wrong.

As explained in the last chapter, focusing on *what* leads you to a solution. Focusing on *who* does nothing more than drain your energy.

Forming good habits

Essentially, you are going through a learning process, and the more you do it, the easier it becomes. The more you learn about your hair, face shape and what suits you, the more effortless any consultation you have with your hairdresser will become. Remember, however, that your hairdresser is not a mind reader. Even if you have reached the point where you have a style that suits your hair, face and even the rest of your body, if something is bothering you, tell your hairdresser.

Although your hair is not alive, it is attached to you, and you are very much alive. As a living organism, you are changing all the time, and for all you know, something could have taken place on the inside since your last visit to change the texture or behaviour of your hair – a shift in hormones or balance of nutrients, for instance.

Getting into the habit of being open with your hairdresser and talking about any changes you have noticed with your hair – good and bad – and letting them share any changes they may have spotted is another way of moving towards hair happiness.

Hair happiness is not something that happens by chance. It happens by design, so we all have the potential to achieve it. If we make a conscious commitment to changing our attitudes and behaviours and, of course, to following the guidance in this book, we have it within us to become whomever we want to be.

You don't have to make grand gestures. You can start by taking small, manageable steps each day, which will result in continuous improvement. It can be hard to make big adjustments, leaving you disheartened, but adjusting to little changes and turning them into helpful habits is easy.

Let's consider some different approaches to managing change.

We all have it in us

According to the bell of achievement (commonly known as the bell curve), illustrated in the diagram below, only a small proportion of us will ever achieve our full potential (interpreted as excellent performance rather than meeting expectations). We disagree. We all have unlimited potential, and any one of us can unleash ours – starting with our hair. The problem is that most of us, often through no fault of our own, lack the will or the know-how to reach our fullest potential. Furthermore, reaching our fullest potential means moving out of our comfort zone. As humans, we like comfort. It makes us feel safe. We achieve a certain level of success and are happy if we haven't had to feel discomfort in the process. Why push further if it makes us uncomfortable? We can tell you why: if you don't, you won't experience all that life has to offer. We can help you do that.

Begin by achieving hair happiness, and you can go on to achieve in all areas of your life.

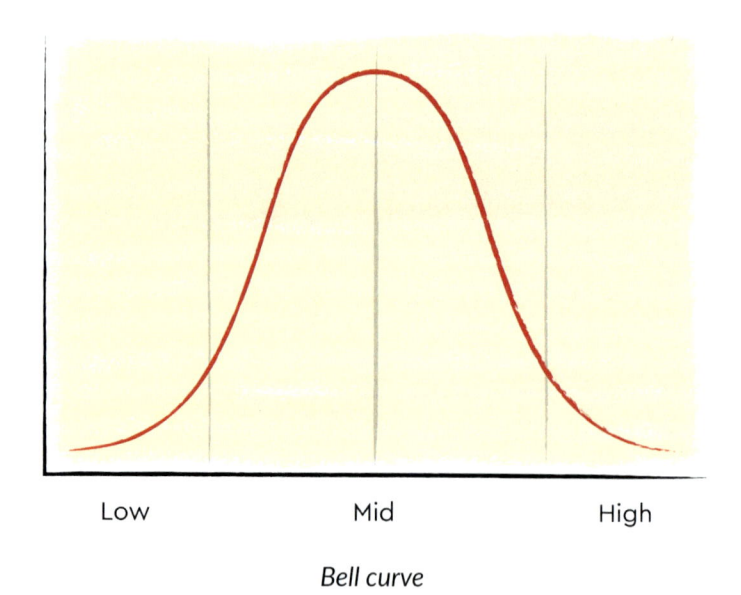

Low   Mid   High

Bell curve

Never stop learning

We must be prepared to learn and develop on an ongoing basis. This doesn't necessarily mean sitting in a classroom, reading a book, listening to a podcast or watching a video tutorial on our phones. It means making an effort to improve every day, no matter how small. It can be as little as asking why instead of taking what we've been told at face value, or consciously refocusing our minds away from any negativity we may feel on waking and towards what we are grateful for. It may be taking a moment to focus our attention away from our busy minds to how we are feeling inside, to connect with our body.

How we choose to experience and embrace every single one of our emotions is our choice. If we choose to interpret our emotions in a way that means we harbour negative feelings and entertain the limiting beliefs that generate them, that's on us. In fact, wherever we end up in life is a direct consequence of the choices we've made.

We can start by teaching you something now. A whopping 95% of our behaviour is habit.[7] Make as much of it good habit as you can.

What are emotions?

It is a word we use all the time, but what exactly are emotions? Emotions are a form of energy in motion, experienced as sensations in the body, and are triggered unconsciously in the here and now. This makes them distinct from feelings. These are generated by conscious thought and can be recalled later and altered depending on whether we change our perception of them. Nevertheless, the terms are used interchangeably.

They are, however, interconnected; our thoughts can influence our emotions and vice versa. Knowing this distinction is important, as a single emotion can trigger different feelings depending on a person's state of mind.

For instance, two people walk into a salon. Both sense their stomach clenching and their heart racing as they experience anticipation. For one, however, that emotion translates into a feeling of dread, as they feel intimidated by the salon staff and fearful they'll miscommunicate what they want and end up with a hair disaster. The other feels pumped and excited and can't wait to discuss the endless possibilities with their stylist.

In both cases, the emotion is what it is. It cannot be changed. The feeling, however, is dependent on the mindset of the person.

Honeymoon period

Starting to change is easy, but how do we keep going? It is human nature to feel energised and optimistic at the start of any change we put in motion – you only have to consider the phrase 'honeymoon period'. Our enthusiasm will, however, likely wane if the change we desire isn't forthcoming or we have a setback, or if we achieve the level of change we were hoping for and then start coasting. As the sigmoid curve in the diagram below shows, our progress then tapers off.

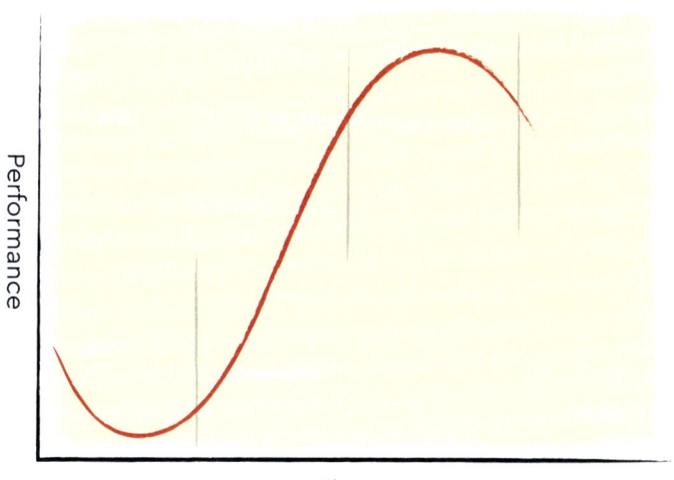

Sigmoid curve

Continuous success is not an accident. To keep improving, you need to take action. If not, the gains you've made level off and you may even start heading in the opposite direction. If what you have been doing is no longer working, look at what you can change. Your hairdresser? Your mindset? Your communication style? Your behaviours? Only you can decide.

> **Sigmoid curve**
>
> The sigmoid curve was developed by Charles Handy to illustrate a company's financial performance (vertical axis) over time (horizontal axis). It is featured in his book, *The Age of Paradox*, although a similar concept had been used in the study of biology since the time of Darwin.[8]
>
> At 365 Day Hairdressing, we decided to apply the concept to skills acquisition and made an intriguing discovery. Whether it's haircutting or learning to play an instrument, the values were equal. Acquisition follows the same curve regardless of the skill. What's more, this proved to be the case in all thirty-two countries where we trained hairdressers, demonstrating the universal applicability of the sigmoid curve in skills acquisition.
>
> As you can see, we have taken the concept a step further and applied it to behaviour change.

Take small steps

As we have said, it's by taking little steps and making small changes each day that big things happen. Being prepared to make changes and try something new will allow you to continuously improve. The saying we often shared when training hairdressers and salon owners across the world sums it up perfectly: 'By the inch, it's a cinch; by the yard, it's hard.'

Progress is also easier when you manage expectations, as we have recommended you do with your hairdresser. You can start each day on a positive note but be realistic – some days will be harder than others. Remember, though, any hard days will pass and in the words of Leslie, 'The wonder of yesterday is whatever we didn't like is behind us.'

In a nutshell, you continue making progress by forming habits to help you continue to move forward. You may not always feel like you are making progress, but as the 'Continuous Improvement' diagram shows, if you continue taking steps and making small changes or adjustments, you will move forwards. There will inevitably be adjustment periods as you make changes and grasp something new, denoted by the troughs in the graph, but it will nevertheless lead to ongoing growth.

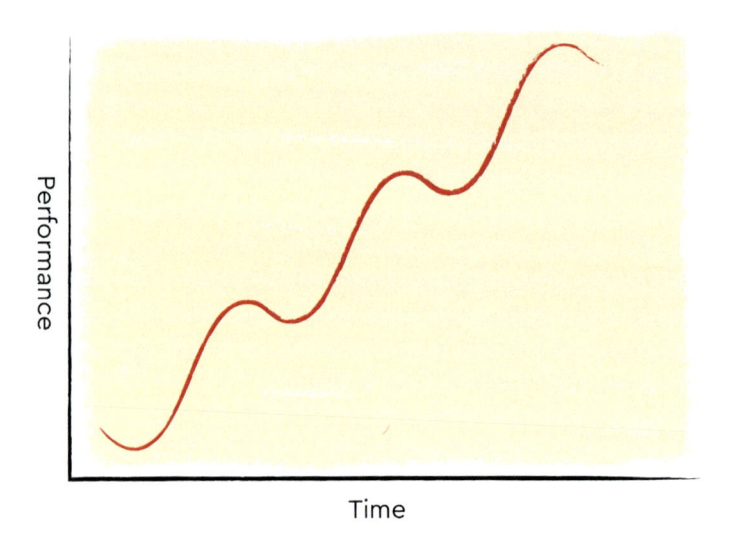

Continuous improvement

Never forget the bigger goal

A word of caution. While taking the smaller steps, be mindful not to forget the bigger goal of hair happiness – this will help you find solutions rather than get bogged down with the daily challenges and dilemmas you will inevitably face.

Over to you

Applying what we have covered in this chapter, what small step can you take first to improve the outcome of your next hair appointment? Do you need to better manage your expectations of what the hairdresser can do for you? Do you need to raise your own expectations? To not settle? Do you need to become better at asking for what you want? To be more curious and assume less?

You could try the following ideas:

- Make a short bullet point list of your likes, dislikes and wishes for your next haircut to use as an aide-memoire.

- Set an incentive (a small treat) to encourage yourself to ask why if you are not sure of something the hairdresser says, or to be more open minded if something they do doesn't fit with your idea of how things should happen.

- Do a five-to-ten-minute meditation/quiet reflection on what's driven your expectations in the past and what you can do to change. Be curious!

To improve your life beyond your hair, you could try these steps:

- Switch negative thoughts to positive ones on waking. For instance, if you are nervous on the morning of your next hair appointment, instead of dreading it, focus on how you will feel walking out with a great haircut you love. Or, if you were frustrated with your hairdresser last time, think about the positive steps you could take to influence a positive outcome. Timing is important, as there is a short window on waking when your brain is at its most suggestible to new ways of thinking.

- Engage in simple activities on waking, such as mindful stretching or breathing for a couple of minutes to help prolong this optimal waking state. Or do a backward countdown.

- If the above suggestions don't sit comfortably, as an alternative, spend a few quiet minutes outside or looking out of the window.

- Before falling asleep, reflect on what you are grateful for.

- Throughout the day, be more curious – ask yourself and others questions.

- Keep learning. It doesn't need to be anything big, just try something new – a new recipe, a new book, a new podcast, a new exercise, a new route to work.

- Stop settling – you are worth more. Encourage yourself to do a task to a higher standard than you usually would, speak up for yourself (or someone else) and ask for more if you believe you deserve more. If you are prone to self-criticism, be kind to yourself. Don't beat yourself up if you don't manage on the first attempt. Simply trying is taking the first step.

- Stop putting yourself last; if the people around you fail to accept this, perhaps it is a sign they might wish to engage in some introspection of their own. Treat people how you would want to be treated – be kind and considerate – but give yourself permission to put yourself first. You don't need to respond to emails, texts, messages or phone calls right away. You don't always need to be switched on and available. If it's not an emergency, what's the worst that can happen? Someone gets annoyed. That's their choice.

Learning checklist

- Communication is only as good as the expectations that underpin it.

- Having the right expectations will help you form a successful relationship with your hairdresser. Remember that it takes mutual effort.

- Forming a successful relationship with your hairdresser happens by design.

- You have to work at it by forming good habits – having the right expectations, understanding what is and isn't realistic and using that as a framework to communicate what you want but also what isn't working and determining how to remedy it.

- Build good habits to achieve hair happiness and you can go on to achieve in other areas of your life.

- Progress won't be in a straight line. There will be periods when you sense you are advancing with ease and times when you feel you are going backwards, but if you continue taking small steps, and are willing to make changes, learn new things and keep your mind on the bigger picture, you will keep making progress. Make a start by having a go at the suggestions in the lists above.

What's next?

You should now be clear on what you can reasonably expect from your hairdresser and how to address and manage your expectations. Next, we'll look at the steps you should take to ensure you have a brilliant hair experience every visit and every day in between, starting with making sure you know your own hair.

6
Get Ready

Before we move on to how you can ensure you have a brilliant experience the next time you visit the salon, or have your hairdresser visit you, we want to pause to give you a quick tutorial on hair. You know your hair is important, but how much do you know about it really? We will show you how to prepare for your next encounter with your hairdresser the smart way.

Starting with why we have hair, we will then look at your hair's structure and take you through the main types before showing you how to spot damage and its causes and what you can do to prevent it in the future.

Why is this important? Does it even matter? Yes. You will be better equipped to spot damage and take steps before even setting foot in the salon or wherever you see your hairdresser. Once there, it will help provide context to your conversations with your hairdresser about styles and aftercare. Your discussions will be better informed and have more depth, setting you up for greater hair happiness. Let's start with the basics.

What is hair and why do we have it?

We are covered in hair. You might have to have a long, hard look to spot it, but you will find hair growing in some form or other on most parts of your body.

Our hair's primary function is to protect our body, whether preserving heat – in the case of the hair on our heads or skin – or preventing dust or other foreign bodies from making their way in, which is why we have nose hairs and eyelashes. Our lashes are not just there to make our eyes pretty.

As you have learned in this book, however, the hair on our heads plays a central role in how we look, which impacts our happiness – whether we like it or not. Let's take a look inside our hair.

Every one of the 100,000 or so hairs most of us have on our heads is made up of two parts: the follicle and the shaft.

The follicle is where your hair starts its life and begins to grow. You may have heard hair being referred to as dead – in fact, we described it as such in Chapter 3 – but the hair cells within the follicle are, in fact, alive and are nourished by blood vessels surrounding them under the skin. It is why you feel pain when you pluck a hair out and why your diet can impact your hair health.

Did you know that follicle shape plays a role in whether your hair is curly, wavy or straight? We will reveal more about this as we take you through the main types of hair in the next section.

The shaft is the part of your hair you can see, and here, you would be correct in thinking it is dead. One thing that makes hair so fascinating is that once it has grown above the skin's surface, the cells in it are no longer living, which is why, unlike waxing (ouch!), having your hair cut isn't a painful experience. The shaft is formed of the following four layers, except in hair that is naturally blond and fine:

1. **The medulla** is the innermost layer and is most commonly found in darker and grey hair, but,

interestingly, it is never found in naturally blond and fine hair. Even more intriguing is that it doesn't appear to have any sort of function.

2. **The cortex** is the middle layer and makes up most of the hair shaft, which, along with the medulla, when present, houses the pigmentation cells, known as melanin, that dictate the colour of our hair. Keeping the hair cortex in good shape is essential for strong, healthy hair.

3. **The cuticle** is the outer layer and plays a fundamental role in protecting the inner layers and making your hair look good. Formed of scales – don't worry, we are not descended from reptiles – the cuticle acts like our hair's armour. In healthy hair, these scales lie flat against one another, giving it its shine, but they also make sure nothing breaks through into the cortex. They are flexible when healthy, and this is where your hair gets its bounce. The size of the scales can vary between hair types, which is why some types appear more naturally shiny than others.

4. **The cell membrane complex** provides another layer of protection between the outside world and the cortex.

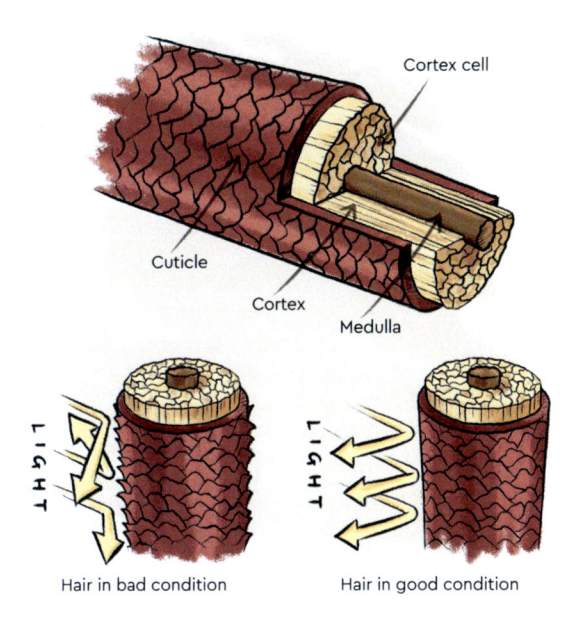

The three layers of the hair and healthy versus damaged hair

Know your type of hair

There are three main types of hair: straight, curly/wavy and coily. The difference essentially comes down to follicle shape, but there are other factors.

Straight hair

Straight hair grows from **round follicles**. It tends to grow **more quickly** than other hair types – or at least gives the illusion of doing so – at about 1.4 centimetres per month. Great if you want long hair, but it is challenging when maintaining a shorter style. That's where the similarity between straight hair types ends.

In some cases, straight hair can be springy in appearance, where the hair grows **directly upwards** from the scalp. While this gives the impression of volume, such hair can be hard to tame and tricky to style and keep down.

Meanwhile, other variants of straight hair have the **lowest density** of all the hair types – as little as 150 hairs per square centimetre of scalp – making it harder to achieve volume in certain hairstyles.

Straight hair can be **smooth and shiny or frizzy**, and it all comes down to the thickness of the hair and the volume of cuticles on each hair shaft, which influences the hair's porosity.

There are types of straight hair with thicker strands that are **less porous**, smoother and shinier in appearance and more resistant to frizz – the result of more tightly packed scales in the cuticle. Note that we are talking about the volume of scales on the cuticle rather than the volume of hair.

If you have thick, straight hair that happens to have fewer, less tightly packed scales on the cuticle, so **more porous**, it will likely be prone to frizz if you fail to follow an appropriate haircare routine.

The shine may, however, result from straight hair being more prone to **becoming oily**. Where there are no kinks or waves in the hair, it's easier for any oil produced on the scalp to spread down the hair shafts. Furthermore, any oil collected on the shaft of straight hair is more visible; there's nowhere for it to hide.

Curly or wavy hair

This type of hair grows from **oval follicles** and often **extends diagonally** from the scalp, so it will stay flat when tied back or styled.

Often **denser** than the other hair types, curly or wavy hair can reach roughly 220 hairs per square centimetre of scalp. It is, therefore, often relatively easy to achieve volume through styling. On the flip side, the high density makes it heavier than the other types of hair, so you'll need hair products or accessories that allow for greater hold to keep it in place.

At about 1.2 centimetres per month, it has one of the **fastest growth rates**, which is why hair appointments, especially for shorter styles, are recommended every six weeks. This hair frequently has a relatively **high porosity** and can be prone to frizz without an appropriate haircare routine.

Coily hair

Coily hair grows from **elliptical-shaped follicles** and **lies almost parallel to the scalp**. The elongated follicle shape gives the hair a flattened appearance, and the hair strands **grow in a spiral**, twisting round on themselves.

Where the coils are tight, the hair gives the impression of growing **slowly**, less than 1 millimetre per month, which is why you will need braiding and weaving with some types of coily hair to achieve longer styles.

Although coily hair types aren't often that dense – around 190 hairs per square centimetre – the strands can be thick, **making it seem denser** than it is in reality. Like curly hair, coily hair tends to have a **higher porosity**, so it is prone to frizz when a proper haircare routine is not followed.

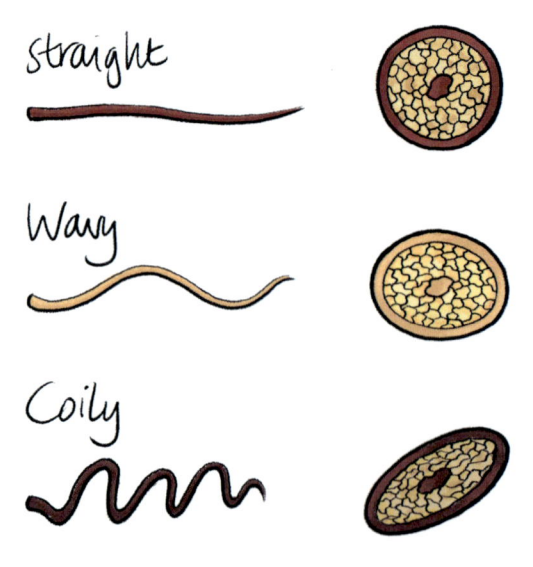

Straight, wavy and coily hair

	Straight	Curly/wavy	Coily
Follicle shape	Round	Oval	Elliptical
Density	Varies but can go as low as 180 per square cm of scalp	Varies but can reach as much as 220 per square cm of scalp	Varies but can go as low as 190 per square cm of scalp
Growth – amount	As much as 1.4 cm per month	Average 1.2 cm per month	0.9 cm per month
Growth – direction from scalp	Varies from diagonal to straight up	Diagonal	Parallel
Considerations	Many variations, from light and springy and hard to tame to thick and prone to frizz. This hair is more oily than other types.	Can be heavier with higher density, requiring stronger hair ties and products. High porosity makes it prone to frizz.	Hair weaving and extensions are an option with some variants of this hair due to slow growth.

Hair health

It is important to know the signs of healthy and unhealthy hair.

Healthy hair:

- Is shiny and smooth
- Has good elasticity – it has a bounce to it that remains all day
- Detangles easily
- Doesn't frizz at the first sign of moisture
- Doesn't break easily
- Depletes by a few strands each day but not en masse

Signs that your hair needs some TLC are obvious: it's lost its va-va-voom, bounce and sheen, or it's started to feel dry and thin out – rather like the pot plant in your living room that you've forgotten to water.

Why does my hair feel dry and brittle?

No matter your hair type, if cracks start forming in the cuticle, your hair will feel coarse and brittle.

Once the cuticle starts to crack, the scales on its surface will begin to lift away from the hair shaft, giving your damaged hair a frizzy appearance. At this point, it also becomes prone to knots and tangling, where the hair is less supple and the strands no longer lie smoothly against one another. Cracked cuticles are also to blame for your hair looking dull, as light always reflects more easily off smooth hair.

Over time, these cracks eventually expose the inner part of your hair, the cortex, where the worst damage can occur, and your hair starts breaking or 'falling out'.

Once your hair is damaged, it can get trapped in a vicious cycle. Damaged hair is prone to further harm because once the cuticle is compromised, your hair will steadily become drier and more brittle, to the point it takes little for it to break off, or it becomes so stretched – by more than twice its original length – that it cannot spring back into shape. This differs from hair elasticity, whereby healthy hair can stretch by about 30% of its original length but easily springs back, giving your hair bounce.

The key is not to let your hair get damaged in the first place. Choosing the right products to protect it when styling sits at the heart of this, and we will come to this later in this chapter and the book. If your hair does become damaged, take action as soon as you spot the first signs. If left, hair stretchiness and brittleness can, in turn, lead to the following complications:

- **Increased porosity:** Your hair has difficulty retaining any oils and moisture it absorbs, so it is perpetually dry.

- **Hair shaft swelling:** Moisture (often from excessive air-drying or sleeping on wet hair) gets into the cell membrane complex – the layer of hydration-creating lipids between the cuticle and the cortex – and causes it to swell. Continued swelling and shrinking of the hair shaft causes it to lose elasticity, making it more vulnerable to breakage.

- **Fractured hair fibres (split ends):** Because your hair grows from the root, it typically splits at the ends – these are the oldest part, so they are most vulnerable – but breakage can happen further up the hair.

- **Damage to your scalp:** Your hair follicles become inflamed, especially where hair is being pulled and stretched, although your follicles can get damaged for other reasons – poor nutrition being one, getting clogged with hair products, another. Damaged hair follicles can result in hair loss or thinning. We'll touch a bit more on hair loss below.

What causes damage?

More than you might imagine. The obvious culprits are washing, styling and straightening.

Where your hair brushes against your clothing, however, or is stuffed under a hat or confined under other headwear, it can become damaged over time – think of the friction. Exposure to cold and hot weather, as well as windy, dry and humid conditions, also plays its part.

Daily wear and tear from all the above causes the damage to the cuticle that we mentioned earlier. Some causes, of course, are more harmful than others:

- **Heat:** Whether from straighteners, heated tongs, your hairdryer or sun exposure, heat can cause untold damage to your hair. Heat forces the cuticles to lift, as described above, exposing the cortex, which, when damaged, leaves your hair brittle and prone to breakage.
- **Lightening:** Hydrogen peroxide when mixed with bleach acts in two ways that can damage your hair. It dissolves the melanin found in the medulla and cortex, removing the original colour. To gain access to the melanin in the cortex, it weakens the keratin in the cuticle by making it swell, which forces the scales to lift. What's more, the keratin in the cuticle is no longer as robust as it was, leaving it vulnerable to further damage from other sources, such as heat.
- **Colouring:** While not as harmful as bleaching, dyeing your hair with permanent dyes can also damage it. Semi-permanents less so. Ingredients

in the dye, such as ammonia, make openings in the cuticle by causing the scales to lift, allowing colour from the dye to penetrate the hair shaft. The hair then swells, closing any openings and trapping the colour inside. Repeated changes to the hair from regular dyeing lead to damage over time, leaving it porous and brittle.

> **Green hairdressing**
>
> When talking about heat and chemicals, it would be remiss of us not to reflect on what the industry is doing to become more sustainable.
>
> For a growing number of us, hair happiness involves choosing salons or hairdressers that are committed to eco-friendly practices. These include using more energy-efficient appliances and techniques, saving water, reducing waste, recycling, and switching to environmentally friendly products.
>
> Every hairdresser and salon should do their bit, no matter how small, to make the world we live in a healthier, happier place.

How to repair and work with damaged hair

We have lots at our disposal to repair damaged hair. In fact, more than at any other time.

GET READY

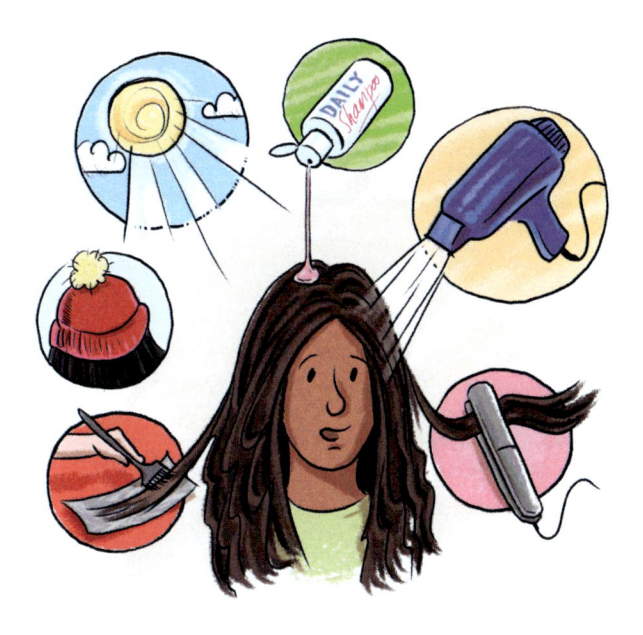

Common causes of hair damage

Your hairdresser will be able to advise you on the right products, for instance. We have included a product and tool tutorial in Chapter 10, but here are some good habits you can develop at home before your next visit:

- **Shampoo your scalp:** Healthy hair starts with a healthy scalp, so focus your shampooing efforts there. Ever noticed your hairdresser giving what feels like a good head massage when washing your hair? They are, in fact, giving your scalp a good wash.

- **Condition those cuticles:** Just to be clear, not the ones surrounding your nails! Focus your conditioner use on the lengths of your hair, where the cuticle is most vulnerable.

- **Comb with care:** Running a comb through your hair when wet to remove tangles and knots might seem like the easier option – but stop. Dragging your comb through wet hair is damaging, as the wetter your hair is, the more vulnerable it is to becoming stretched. Instead, apply a detangling leave-in conditioner and gently comb from the ends up to the roots when your hair is wet. You can also use a high-quality boar bristle brush – more on brushes in Chapter 10.

- **Be patient:** As with combing, towel-dry and then air-dry your hair if you have time until it is mostly dry (about three-quarters) before reaching for your hairdryer.

- **Good nutrition:** Eating plenty of protein and essential fatty acids, particularly omega-3s, are great ways of keeping your hair healthy from the inside. You can find essential fatty acids in flax seeds, chia seeds, walnuts, soybeans, tofu and leafy vegetables, such as broccoli, as well as in fatty fish, such as tuna and salmon. Great sources of protein include fish, chicken, eggs and soy products.

If your hair is damaged, choose a suitable haircut. The style your hairdresser recommends will depend on your hair type and other factors, such as growth patterns and your face shape, which we will come to later, but layering to add texture is a common technique to overcome hair damage. Your hairdresser will also recommend products and home styling that can hide the appearance of damaged hair while it is healing.

Ageing gracefully

Many of us, particularly women or those identifying as female, choose to dye our hair to cover those pesky grey hairs the moment they inevitably appear. What if you decide to embrace your natural hair colour as it gradually shifts towards grey, silver or white? Or what if you are unable to dye your hair for whatever reason? How do you showcase your maturing hair in all its natural glory?

Hair turns grey through loss of pigment as we age. Either the pigment is no longer produced by the follicle, which is the case with most hair types, or, in red hair, the pigment fades – this is why this hair type turns yellow and then eventually white, rather than grey. This loss of pigment will happen to us all to a greater or lesser degree, but do we need to hide it?

Instead of covering the grey, what's stopping you from going for all-out coverage? These days, hairdressers have many tools and techniques at their disposal to showcase your natural grey, bringing out the depth and shine in this much-underrated colour and giving you a look that is elegant, sophisticated or distinguished, depending on what you're aiming for.

The decision to embrace your grey can feel like a watershed moment, so if you need time, take it. Discuss it with your hairdresser. It's not a decision you should rush or take lightly, as it encompasses so much more than choosing to have blond, red, brown or black hair. It is about leaning into and accepting that you are growing older. If you are thinking about embracing your grey (or white) hair, consider the following questions: why is it important? How do you think it will make you feel? How would you feel if you decided not to?

Hair loss is another sign of ageing, although it can happen for other reasons. When it does occur, it can really impact how you feel about yourself. Your hairdresser can help. Talk to them about your options. Ask for recommendations of specialist clinics. Hair loss shouldn't exclude you from hair happiness.

Measure twice, cut once

Some hairdressers will offer a pre-appointment consultation to assess your hair type and its condition along with other needs, such as your lifestyle, which, again, we will cover more in the next chapter. They will most likely take you through a lookbook, too, which will help you visualise any style you discuss. The more prepared they are before they reach for the scissors, the better.

If your hairdresser can't… find one who can, for this is not a step you should miss. Any good hairdresser and salon should be offering pre-appointment consultations, of course. It may not be your hairdresser, but a junior team member, as delivering these consultations can form part of their training and skills development.

Otherwise, maybe you can find a hair coach to step into the breach, at least when understanding your hair type and its care needs. Some are trained trichologists. That being the case, they can advise you on your scalp health.

We recommend, however, that you exercise caution. Ideally, for consistency, you should work with your hairdresser end to end, or, if they cannot, members of the same salon team, to ensure you do not receive conflicting advice, which can be worse than no advice.

AI – blessing or curse?

Like in other industries, AI is finding its way into hairdressing, whether as a tool to create efficiencies – for instance, streamlining booking processes – or a solution to previously unsolved challenges. There has been talk of using AI to mix hair colours and similar, although there is currently little confidence in its effectiveness.

When applied to something like building a customer's confidence to go for a new look by

> showing them on-screen what it could look like on them first, AI has had a warmer reception, but that's probably because it would still involve human input.
>
> It has the potential to make pre-appointment consultations the norm. Does it have the potential to show clients what their hair could look like if they continue to follow damaging practices, or, better still, how great it could look if they begin following good haircare habits? In other words, showing them hair happiness before the fact – how powerful that would be.

If you decide to try a hair coach, choose carefully. Like hairdressers, they will vary in quality, but a good one should provide tailored advice between visits, and if you can see them in person, they should be able to give you hands-on help, including developing the good habits we shared above.

Still, we maintain that your hairdresser should offer this consultation, and if they are telling you they don't have the time, it's not true. As hairdressers, we can always find the time. If it is not practical to change your hairdresser right now, make sure you are prepared and use the information in this chapter and the next to come up with questions to ask them at the start of your appointment. Either way, the goal is that you head into any pre-appointment consultation or hair appointment far more informed.

Learning checklist

- Hair's primary function is protection, but its role goes far beyond this.
- Knowing how hair is structured will help you understand how to keep it healthy.
- There are three types of hair: straight, curly and coily. Each hair type has different features and care needs.
- Although there are differences between the three hair types, there are common factors to consider when caring for hair – at its heart good haircare is about forming better habits around haircare, mindset and nutrition.
- There are also common factors that can damage hair, but there are simple ways to avoid damage – again, it comes down to forming good habits.
- The pre-appointment consultation can play a key role in assessing your hair health.

What's next?

Now you've got to grips with your hair, and how to keep it healthy, we will take you step by step through how to make the most of your salon visit.

7
More Than A Pretty Face

Preparation is key, as any good hairdresser will tell you. In fact, it is essential for achieving hair happiness. For this reason, we will continue to help you get ready for your next haircut by enlisting your hairdresser's help and encouraging you to consider the bigger picture. We will show you why you should be considering more than you might realise ahead of your next haircut.

Now you are aware of just how amazing your hair is – who knew science could be so interesting – we want to cast your mind back to the Ebbinghaus illusion, the diagram in Chapter 1 that shows how the size and shape of something is clearly influenced by whatever we place next to it.

Greater than the sum of your parts

You can use your hairstyle to make the most of your face shape, but at the same time, your face shape should influence the hairstyle you and your hairdresser settle on – yes, once again, choosing your hairstyle should be a team effort.

Your hair, face and, indeed, the rest of you are greater than the sum of your parts, as are you and your hairdresser. We recommend you use this as the basis for any discussions with your hairdresser once you are in the chair – or at a pre-appointment consultation if they offer these. We will continue our discussion on the benefits of a pre-appointment consultation in more depth later. Either way, the handy chart below will help you have a far more informed discussion, especially if you take a good look at it at home beforehand. Not sure you have time? Use the tips we share in the book to develop the habit of making time. You deserve it.

We've said it before, and we'll keep saying it – both you and your hairdresser should play a role in the decisions you make about your hair. Listen to whatever your hairdresser has to say, but don't defer to them. Remember the model and Britain's Finest Hair Ambassador in Chapter 4? Never tell them 'Do what you want.' We also have a cautionary tale coming up in Chapter 9.

Only you can know what you want, and, as discussed in Chapter 3, there are many drivers to this. You need to share what you want with your hairdresser, and understanding what suits your hair type, face and body shape will help. All the same, while you shouldn't defer to them, understand they have a wealth of professional expertise and knowledge they can bring to the table that you should be open to taking on board.

In recommending a style, your hairdresser should be attempting to bring out the good and flatter the not-so-good. Despite what some might like to think, no single human being walking this earth is perfect; we all have a feature or two that need flattering. What's more, a good hairdresser will recommend a hairstyle that does this wonderfully, and, for your part, understanding why they might be championing a particular hairstyle will make settling on one that will result in hair happiness that much easier.

For instance, you might have beautiful, sculpted cheekbones but a nose that is perhaps a little too much on the prominent side, in which case the hairdresser might suggest a hairstyle that will bring out your cheekbones but will add volume at the back, which will help to balance out the prominence of your nose.

Face shape

It is important to know what your face shape is. Getting down to the nitty-gritty, we have one of six main face shapes, all with varying characteristics and flattered by different hairstyles. Use the following charts to determine yours.

Face shapes

	Oval	Square	Round	Heart	Rectangular	Diamond
Characteristics	• Face length longer than width • Jawline marginally narrower than hairline	• Jawline and hairline are same width • Angular jawline	• Width and length of face are the same, like a circle	• Wide hairline tapering down into a narrow jawline with prominent cheekbones	• Much like oval but chin is longer	• Jawline and hairline are same width • Cheekbones are wider
Goal of hairstyle	• Most styles work with this face shape, so focus on other factors such as lifestyle, whether the client wears glasses, etc	• Create illusion of longer face • Possibly soften jawline	• Create illusion of longer face	• Soften widow's peak • Strengthen jawline	• Create illusion of shorter, broader face • Soften jawline	• Highlight cheeks and eyes • Soften angular features

Facial hair (men*)	• Most beard styles work with an oval face • For those who want the illusion of a more sculptured face, balbo, long stubble or a full beard work well	• Round or triangular shaped to counterbalance square jaw • Styles that lengthen and soften the jaw – goatee, circle or balbo beards, or simply stubble	• Beards that are shorter at the sides and longer on the chin will lengthen the face. Goatee or balbo, etc • Moustaches draw attention to centre of face • Avoid sideburns	• Need to avoid softening of face • Rather than full beard – stubble and sideburns • Shorter beards that won't swamp your face	• Beards that are shorter on the bottom and longer on the sides • Accentuate strong jawline	• Avoid pointy • Rounded and blunt edges work best Shorter styles best but opt for goatee or round if you want length
Eye wear	• Most frame shapes will suit	• Angular frames work well against well-defined jawline so glasses with geometric shapes for bold looks or softer oval frames for subtle looks	• Glasses that lengthen and provide contrast to the roundness and softness of the face • For instance, rectangular glasses	• Most frame shapes will suit	• 'Taller' lenses to shorten the face • Rounder frames soften features	• Rounder frames to soften features

Assigned male at birth or identifying as male

Are you surprised? Is your current hairstyle one that flatters your face shape, judging by the chart? If not, do some research into hairstyles that suit your face shape ahead of your next hair appointment.

You have no doubt heard about how symmetrical faces are deemed more attractive, but do genuinely symmetrical faces exist? The answer is no. We are all less than perfect to some degree, and it's one of the hairdresser's greatest gifts to be able to help you showcase your assets and draw attention away from any imperfections.

You are so much more than a pretty – or handsome – face. When considering your hair beyond your face shape, you will need to bear a number of things in mind.

Body shape

What you see in the hairdresser's mirror is only part of the picture. Your hair must complement your whole body and not just your face. In Chapter 9, we will give you a tip on how to ensure your hairdresser takes your whole body into account, with the help of the aforementioned cautionary tale.

Lifestyle

As explained in Chapter 3, your job or profession and what you do in your leisure time should play a role in your choice of hairstyle. Although we encourage hairdressers not to put you on the spot by asking you about your profession but rather to find out whether you have any professional or social demands that could influence your choice of hairstyle, there is no harm in asking yourself that question.

Think about what you do for a living and how you spend your time outside work. How much free time and disposable income do you have? Do you need a low-maintenance haircut, or can you devote reasonable time to styling your hair each morning or before an evening out? If you are leaning towards a shorter or longer style due to your lifestyle, which length do your hair type, face and body shape best suit? Which best suits the time you have available to spend on your hair?

Be clear about how much time you have available for the haircut, but don't forget to consider how much time you have available for styling your hair at home or when out and about. Is there scope for you to shift your mindset in this regard? Could a hair coach help you? Do your profession and lifestyle require an off-the-shoulder look (either in cut or style), or can you let your hair hang loose (and long)? How often can you visit the salon? How often do you want to? Some hairstyles, such as the pixie cut, while easy to manage on a day-to-day basis will involve regular visits to the hairdresser to keep them looking fresh and avoid the dreaded pyramid hair (especially a risk for people with thick hair).

Here are some low-maintenance options.

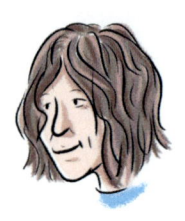

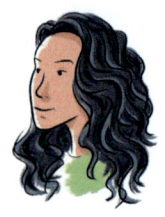

Female

- Shaggy bob, lob etc
- Cuts with long layers
- Any cut that makes styling easy and allows you to go longer between haircuts
- Simple styling products can add texture and hold
- Or go completely natural

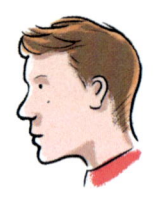

Male

- Short, back and sides
- Cut that requires little to no styling and is easily maintained with a haircut every few weeks
- Simple styling products can add texture and hold
- Or go completely natural

Life stage

What's going on in your life that could impact your hair? We touched on this earlier to help you understand your motivations towards your hair and the style you select, but, again, your health, and hormonal and other changes, will impact your hair. Do you spend time caring for others, or are you a free agent? Are you pregnant or going through the menopause? Is there a family history of premature balding or going grey? Do you have health conditions, or are you undergoing treatments that might affect your hair? Even if you think something is unlikely to impact your hair, it's worth mentioning, as your hairdresser might know otherwise. Once again, you are the expert on you, and your hairdresser is the expert on hair, and by playing it right, you can make a formidable team. If you are facing significant health issues or life-stage changes, bringing a hair coach onto your team could also be an option. Going back to the previous chapter, changes in your hair as you age or go through pregnancy or medical treatment will impact its vulnerability to damage, so you need to bear this in mind.

As explained earlier, we strongly encouraged every hairdresser trained in the 365 Day Hairdressing system to meet and greet every client at reception and to take note of more than their hair, so why not follow suit and make sure you have considered the bigger picture?

Speak up

As discussed in Chapter 4, a good or bad haircut can result more from communication than technique. Although we encourage the hairdressers that we train to greet you and ask plenty of questions, not all hairdressers do. This may signal it's time to change your salon or hairdresser, but we appreciate there may be various reasons why this isn't an option for everyone.

If the situation requires it, take the initiative. Talk to your hairdresser. Using the prompts we have given you above, have something prepared to tell them about what you do for work and leisure, or, indeed, anything that's going on in your life that could be relevant to your hair. You might not think it relevant, but let the hairdresser be the judge of that.

To help you communicate this to your hairdresser, why not create a backstory for your hair ready to share with them. A hair backstory will facilitate more effective communication between you and your hairdresser. It will give you a means of directing the conversation if your hairdresser doesn't take the initiative. Here are two examples to help you work out what to say.

Example One: I have always found my hair relatively easy to style when I wear it long. I have to wash it every few days, or it gets greasy. I currently use a high-street brand of shampoo and conditioner to keep my hair clean and nourished. When styling, I use a combination of a hairdryer with a paddle or round hairbrush and hair straighteners, along with mousse and heat protection spray. I wear my hair longer because when I've had it cut short, sections of it stick out at random angles unless I carefully style them into place. I would like shorter hair because I white-water canoe outside work, and it's easier to fit shorter hair under a helmet. Plus, it dries more quickly. Can you recommend a short style that would work for my hair? Can you explain why my hair behaves the way it does when it is short?

Example Two: My hair has always been tricky to style. I have a strange parting, and my hair is not straight, wavy, thick or fine. The best word to describe it is 'in-between'. I regularly dye it blond, as my natural colour is a nondescript mousy brown. My go-to style is shoulder-length with minimal layers. I straighten it daily, as I would rather that than let it have its feeble waves. The regular straightening and bleaching have damaged the hair, which I try to mitigate with serum. The only saving grace of my hair is that I don't need to wash it frequently. I am not happy with my hair as it is. What can you recommend?

In Chapter 9, we will visit, in more detail, the questions your hairdresser should be asking to elicit this information. If you are lucky to have a hairdresser who does, having a backstory prepared will help you answer the questions concisely. It will also give you something to offer to the hairdresser if they haven't taken the initiative and asked those questions, or if this is how you prefer to communicate.

A picture paints a thousand words – the lookbook

Another tool at your and your hairdresser's disposal to help you prepare for your next haircut is a lookbook. Does your hairdresser or salon have one? Have they used one with you to help explain and choose your haircut? If not, then it's high time we get you acquainted.

A lookbook is a tool that helps your hairdresser communicate the type of haircut and style they are recommending and why. At the same time, you can use one to share what you are looking for in a haircut. It is not a tool for finding a hairstyle for the hairdresser to copy.

You don't pick a picture and say 'That's the hairstyle I want.' Instead, your hairdresser will show you three or four pictures which they will use to illustrate and explain why they are proposing a particular hairstyle in terms of texture, length, colour and shape. They will also point out styles to avoid and why. Accordingly, you can use the visuals to share what you like and don't like, what you think will work for your face and body shape and other factors such as lifestyle and stage. This is because you are unique, and your hairstyle should be bespoke to you.

Just as a tailored gown or suit has been made to fit you perfectly, so should the gown or suit you never take off. Ultimately, a lookbook will help you and your hairdresser design a hairstyle specifically for you.

Do you have some hairstyle ideas in mind? If so, why not do it yourself and make up your own lookbook to help explain what you are looking for to your hairdresser.

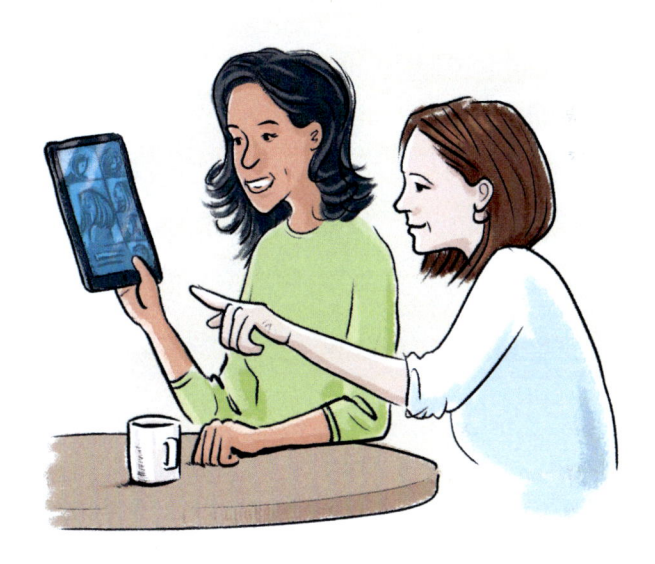

Lookbook consultation

From the hairdresser's perspective, a good lookbook will feature models of all ages unless the salon or your hairdresser targets a specific age group. It will also have sections – for example, short hair, funky hair, mid-length hair, long hair with layers, fringes, bridal hair, men's haircuts etc – and will feature all three hair types that we covered in the last chapter. This will allow your hairdresser to easily locate relevant hairstyles to help illustrate why they are recommending a particular style to you.

A lookbook doesn't have to be a physical book. Your hairdresser might have theirs on a phone or tablet, as can you. Platforms like Pinterest make it easy. What's important is that your hairdresser has a way of showing you pictures to help illustrate why the length, texture of curls or waves (if relevant), or the colour or shape they are recommending will suit you. Likewise, you have a way of showing them what you want, like and don't like. It's easier to explain using visuals than words.

Pre-appointment consultations

We have alluded to pre-appointment consultations thus far but have yet to cover them in detail. Given that they are essential to preparing for your appointment, we will now, bringing together all the points discussed in this chapter.

As we've mentioned before, some salons and hairdressers offer pre-appointment consultations where you can go through a lookbook and discuss what you want. In an ideal world, all should. Ask. It may be that they do, but they offer them only when requested. If they don't, ask if some time can be set aside at the beginning of the appointment for a proper consultation about your hairstyle needs. It's easier if you are getting your hair dyed, as you will need to go in for a patch test forty-eight hours before.

If a pre-appointment consultation is out of the question, this again is where you might benefit from consulting with a hair coach who can advise you on styles, which you can then share with your hairdresser. Of course, this will depend on your available time and budget. Again, we recommend you find a hairdresser who offers an end-to-end service, but we appreciate that factors such as location might not make this easy for everyone. As we touched on earlier, some hairdressers, particularly those not constrained by long-standing, rigid processes in their salon, whether down to how the salon is run or because they are self-employed, are taking the lead in offering remote consultations to prospective clients and to existing clients between cuts. Anything that enhances the client–hairdresser relationship sounds good to us.

If the consultation is a bolt-on to your appointment, we recommend your hairdresser sits with you in a quiet area away from the styling station and any disruptions, if the salon set-up allows. The word 'sit' is key here, as the fact you are both sitting down encourages the consultation to happen on an equal footing (no pun intended). It is a consultation, after all, not the hairdresser telling you what they are going to do or vice versa.

It doesn't need to be long: ten minutes can often suffice. Typically, we tell our clients to bring pictures of them with their favourite and least favourite hairstyles, along with pictures showing examples of hairstyles they love. We ask them about their likes and dislikes and consult them on their face shape and everything else we have covered in this chapter, referring to the lookbook as we go. We even ask clients to bring in their products and styling tools (brushes, tongs, straighteners etc). If you don't need a patch test and it will be a struggle to get in for a ten-minute appointment in person, why not suggest a remote consultation?

The tips and tools we have shared so far and will continue to share in this book will ensure you get the best out of your consultation with your hairdresser. Being prepared for your appointment, either by having a pre-appointment consultation or by making sure you have spent time thinking about what you want and why, will increase the chances of you walking out of the salon at the end of your appointment with a genuine big smile on your face because you have hair happiness.

More often than we'd like, we have clients sit in the chair and say 'I haven't thought about me; I've been so busy I don't quite know what I want.' Even with the best will in the world on our part, they are running the risk of hair unhappiness.

> **Insight from Alison Cooney: On the same page**
>
> A client once asked me for a graduated bob.
>
> 'What do you mean by a graduated bob?' I responded. 'Don't you know?' asked the client, looking puzzled.
>
> 'There are many variations of a graduated bob,' I explained. 'I'd like to confirm we are thinking the same amount of graduation or layering. Something like this?' I said, scrolling through my lookbook on my tablet and stopping on a picture of a model with a bob with layers that graduated sharply from the crown.
>
> 'Oh, no, nothing so severe,' replied the client.
>
> 'What about this then?' I said, scrolling to a picture of a model with a bob that was only lightly graduated at the bottom. 'Perfect,' said the client.
>
> Would we have achieved hair happiness had I not checked we had the same understanding of a graduated bob? Probably not!

More than a snap decision

When you consider everything we have told you so far about hair and its role in your happiness, it is astounding that so many of us have formed the habit of walking into a salon and putting this precious gown or suit we never take off into the hands of a stranger, often with little consultation. It's one of the consequences of the commoditisation of hair services we spoke about in Chapter 2, and it is why we encourage the hairdressers we train to offer free-of-charge, no-commitment, two-way pre-appointment consultations.

It is also why we are asking you to expect more from your hairdresser and/or salon. Selecting who handles your hair should be a considered decision, not a snap one made as you walk down the street or because a friend or someone you follow has posted a great picture of their new hairstyle on Instagram or TikTok. If you do want to use a hairdresser you've come across on social media, aim to have a video consult with them at the least. For those of you in the habit of making a snap decision, you're only choosing the salon, not the hairdresser. Who ends up cutting your hair is often down to timing – whichever hairdresser happens to be available when you walk in or call up for an appointment. Remember, too, that the most accomplished hairdressers in any salon are most likely to be fully booked, so if you decide to simply walk in, it stands to reason that the hairdresser who is available may well not give you or your hair the experience you deserve.

Regardless of how you find yourself in the hairdresser's chair, if you aren't feeling the right chemistry with a particular hairdresser, don't be afraid to say you've changed your mind. We know it is easier said than done, and it is why pre-appointment consultations are so valuable – we can't emphasise enough that you should get into the habit of asking for these – as they come with less expectation and are easier to walk away from should you decide the hairdresser isn't for you. Understand your hair is precious and that you shouldn't put it in the hands of just anyone.

If you are not in a position to change your hairdresser, then make sure you go to the appointment with an understanding of your hair type, face shape, body shape and so on, and that there is a discreet consultation of some kind involving a lookbook – theirs, yours or both.

We know change isn't going to happen overnight, but if one by one each of us starts expecting more from our hairdresser and/or salon, it will eventually become the norm.

Learning checklist

- You can use your hairstyle to make the most of your face shape, but at the same time, your face shape should influence the hairstyle (and beard for those of you who want or have one). Understand yours before heading to your next appointment.

- You are greater than the sum of your parts. Consider the bigger picture – your body shape, for instance.

- Be prepared. Know what you want (and what you don't want) but, equally, be prepared to listen to your hairdresser.

- Consider creating a hair backstory and a lookbook to show your hairdresser.

- Insist on a pre-appointment consultation in some shape or form.

What's next?

Now you are armed and prepared for your hair appointment, we will move on to how to ensure hair happiness once you step into the salon, including how to manage what's running through your head (and the same for your hairdresser) as you set eyes on one another. Even if it's not for the first time.

8
It's Not What You Do, It's The Way That You Do It

By now, you should be incredibly well prepared for your next hair appointment, but what should you consider as you step into the salon or wherever you choose to have your hair cut? How will it help you achieve hair happiness? How can arriving in style set you up for a great hair appointment?

The best version of you

Be yourself, but the best version of you. If you are naturally reserved, don't feel you have to be flamboyant, and vice versa. Authenticity wins through every time. As hairdressers with decades of experience, trust us – we know people.

HAIR HAPPINESS

As we asked when exploring the role of body language in how you communicate earlier in the book, do you stride in with purpose, or do you shuffle in? Think about the messages your body language is giving off. Curling in on yourself and shuffling through the door won't do you any favours. Even the most shy and reserved person can hold their head up, pull their shoulders back and walk into somewhere with purpose. You're still being authentic. You're still you. Just the best version of you.

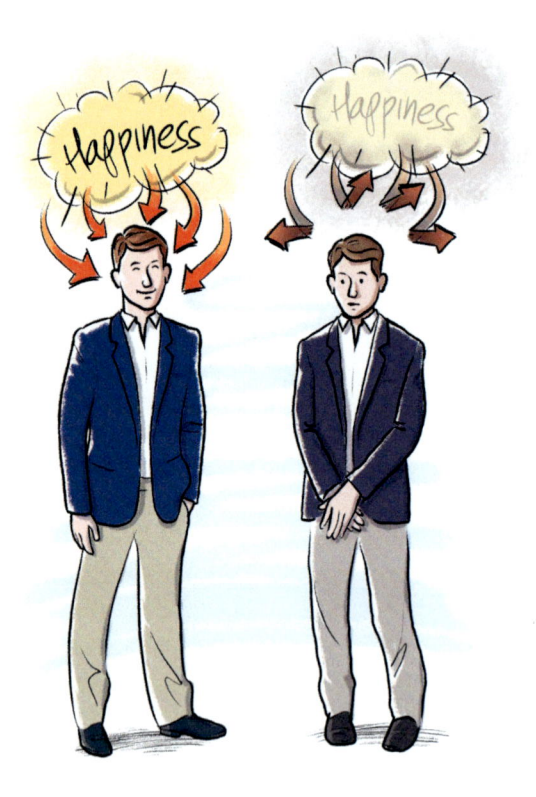

Posture and its role in your happiness

In doing so, you'll naturally feel more confident without trying. You will automatically speak more clearly and with greater assuredness – not least because your improved posture will allow you to breathe more air into your lungs. The greater confidence you feel will, in turn, improve your mood, which will feed an upturn in your hairdresser's mood without them even realising it.

In training hundreds of hairdressers to speak in public, one tip we would give them before going on stage was to stand ramrod straight with their back flush against a wall so as much of their head and body as possible was touching the wall. We then told them to take a few deep breaths, close their eyes and imagine they were about to eat their favourite meal. It worked wonders, particularly in overcoming nerves.

How? Having your back against the wall creates a feeling of safety. Standing helps draw energy downwards, away from where it can feed any anxious thoughts in your mind, allowing you to feel grounded and in the present. Focusing on imagining eating your favourite meal helps generate feel-good hormones – your brain can't tell the difference between what's real and imagined – which also acts to reduce nerves and anxiety.

Others' judgement of you

Why are we telling you this? Because, like everyone else, we hairdressers are prone to that human trait of judgement. Even if we know you well, we will be making judgements based on how you behaved as you walked through our door, which will be reflected in our behaviour towards you. We won't even realise we are doing it. We will be doing it out of habit – our brain's way of saving energy.

Nor will we completely register how we behave on a conscious level. Of course, we are nevertheless responsible for keeping ourselves in check, being aware that we might be making decisions unconsciously, reserving judgement and aiming to be the best versions of ourselves, just as you are. It comes back to the intra- and interpersonal intelligence we spoke about in an earlier chapter.

If *you* want to achieve hair happiness, you need to set the right tone, starting with how you carry yourself as you step into the salon. It will flavour how we perceive you from then on in, from what you say to what you do. If you want us to treat you like the best version of you, then you need to behave that way.

If you have developed a habit of closing yourself off from the world – and there may well be legitimate reasons for this – start small and build up. We know, having worked with thousands of people around the world, that you are far happier when you let others in. Start by simply holding your head up and rolling your shoulders back as you walk through the door, like we said at the beginning of the chapter. You'll find people will want to come into your world because your body language is telling them 'Welcome'. You'll find it so much easier to get the hairstyle you want, especially given the level of two-way communication that we have shown it involves, if you let people in.

How you want to be judged is down to you. You need to take charge.

> **The power of paradigms**
>
> How we view the world and interpret events around us depends on the beliefs we have come to hold, which, in turn, have been formed by our experiences and the people in our lives that have influenced us – otherwise known as a paradigm.
>
> Paradigms are powerful, yet few appreciate the extent of their influence, positive and negative, over the direction our lives take. How you judge others and others judge you is rooted in paradigms.
>
> We all have the power to shift our paradigms. The question is by how much to achieve hair happiness. Only you can answer that.

Your judgement of others

Just as we make subconscious judgements about you, you will do the same about us. Maybe our striking make-up, expertly styled hair or flamboyant nature is intimidating. Don't let it be. You wouldn't want to eat in a dirty, down-at-heel restaurant, so it follows that having your hair cut by a bedraggled-looking hairdresser would hardly inspire confidence.

We are walking advertisements for our skill and expertise, and as much as we'd love to, we can't adapt our hair, dress and make-up to suit every client, so we go with what makes us comfortable and what's authentic to us. We are, by nature, an open, people-loving bunch, which is reflected in how we present ourselves to the world.

It doesn't mean that if you are the quiet or more reserved type, we cannot get along with you. We trained hairdressers in the 365 Day Hairdressing system how to connect with all types of people. On the flip side, you might be more flamboyant than your hairdresser. Reserve judgement, be curious and get to know them, as hair happiness results from you working as a team.

It's why we recommend asking for a pre-appointment consultation. It will give you the chance to discover more about the hairdresser and to decide if you can be a team without having to first commit to them cutting your hair. Like we said in the previous chapter, if it's not offered, speak up and ask for one.

In short, you will subconsciously make a judgement about your hairdresser the moment you first set eyes on them, and vice versa. Hair happiness is contingent on you both being aware of this happening but not acting on it, reserving judgement and being open to discovering who you each truly are, uncoloured by prejudice or assumptions. This also applies when deciding not to work with a hairdresser, as touched on in the previous chapter.

This sounds great, you say, but how do you reserve judgement? Before we get to that, we need to look at why we make judgements.

Why do we make judgements?

When we make judgements, we draw on the assumptions we form about whatever is in front of us, literally or figuratively. We all draw assumptions, form opinions and use them to make decisions without realising it – a process that, for the most part, is an unconscious one. The nature of our assumptions will be based on the values, attitudes and behaviours we have adopted as a result of our life experiences.

Why do we behave this way? As explained in Chapter 4, it is so our brains save energy. Conscious thinking requires energy, so the brain has adapted, developing unconscious cognitive processes to conserve it. This energy-saving technique is called habit-forming, and our brain is resoundingly good at it – we choose just 5% of what we do consciously.[9]

When we are making assumptions and turning them into judgements, it's our brain's way of saving energy. If we want to achieve hair happiness, we need to stop making assumptions – and we mean positive as well as negative assumptions – and get into the habit of reserving judgement instead. Yes, it will mean using more of our brain's energy in the short term but don't worry, there are other ways we can get our brain to save energy, which we'll come to.

How to reserve judgement

We start by becoming more self-aware, tapping into our intrapersonal intelligence to understand what we think and why. Head back to Chapter 5 for some tips on how to do this. We then use this insight to make positive changes to how we think and what we tell ourselves. Over time, we embed those changes as good habits.

Habits can be useful. As we have said, they cut down on the energy the brain uses by reducing how much conscious decision-making we engage in. We can help ourselves by deciding on the good habits we need to adopt and then automating the decisions involved in sticking with those habits.

Like programming, we create rules. For instance, when forming the habit of reserving judgement, you tell yourself that when you encounter someone or

IT'S NOT WHAT YOU DO, IT'S THE WAY THAT YOU DO IT

something new, you are going to move your focus away from any thoughts that pop into your mind or feelings that assert themselves. Instead, you will take the situation at face value as it presents itself in front of you. As we said in Chapter 4, it's like directing your own mental movie.

OK, but how do you get this to stick?

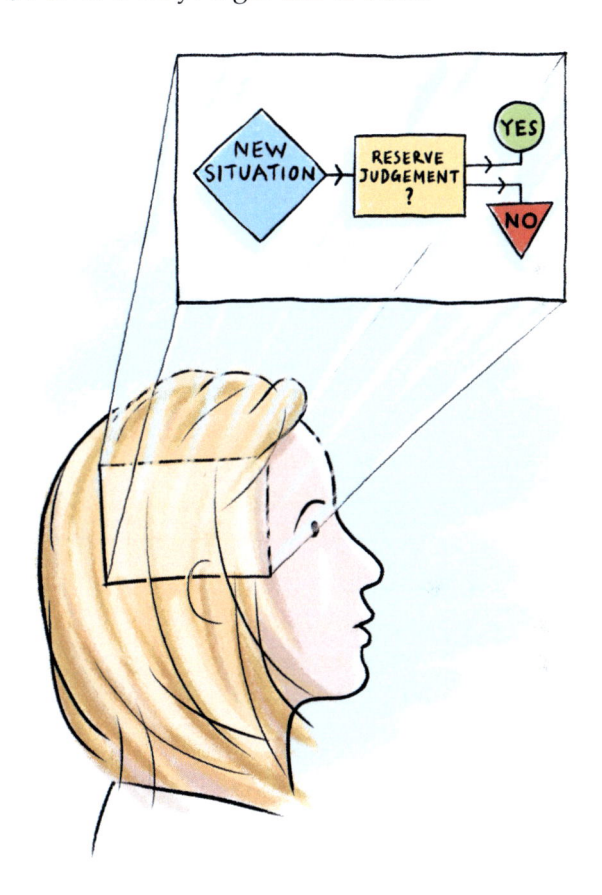

Forming habits

By design and not chance, as we explained in Chapter 5. By really understanding *why* you have acted the way you have in the past and determining why it isn't helpful. By letting go of self-justification: the stories you tell yourself that justify your mistakes and mistaken beliefs and which hold you back and limit you. By taking the time to be curious about how you have come to hold those beliefs and why. These responses will help you stop creating those stories and acting the way you have.

Get your morning D-DOSE

We shared some useful models and tips in Chapter 5, which we hope you have begun to adopt, and we'd like to share another with you now. Taken together, they can all play a role in you becoming the unlimited version of yourself and achieving hair happiness.

Like the others, this latest model is simple but effective. All you have to do is make sure you have your D-DOSE each morning. Make it a rule. Start small with what you think you can easily do, then halve it. Yes, you read that right. Forming new habits is about being consistent, and you are more likely to do something consistently if you maintain interest in it. You will have more success at remaining interested in it if you don't make it too hard. Once it has become second nature, then you can build up.

D-DOSE is your 'smoothie' of daylight, dopamine, oxytocin, serotonin and endorphins, the body's happy chemicals. It's your daily helping of self-love. You can tap into these natural elements in a number of ways:

- Energise yourself through exercise. We are built to move – movement helps our brains form neural pathways, enhancing memory, cognition and, ultimately, our capacity to learn and improve.

- Create the habit of introspection and becoming more conscious and connected to your body with meditation and mindful breathing (or an alternative if you find these triggering[10]).

- Build and nurture social and emotional connections – we are born with the innate ability to do exactly this, and if we harness it by becoming more curious and open-minded, the opportunities are endless. We go so much further when we join forces with others.

We also call this the trilogy of new habits: 'A Life. B Self. C Interdependence.'

For those of you who need it, it's your morning D-DOSE that will give you the courage to step through the salon door with purpose, or to open up to your hairdresser and become a formidable team, or to speak up and say you've changed your mind even if, after reserving judgement and keeping an open mind, you don't feel confident your hairdresser will give you the cut you deserve.

In short, you are in control of how you feel about any situation and, consequently, how you behave. It's the sum of what you perceive, see and think, which, as we trust you now understand, you can become proficient in.

Start your relationship with your hairdresser – or indeed any relationship – on the right foot, or reboot it with an open mind that is free of assumptions. One where you are conscious of any judgements you are making, and you can move to reserve them.

Be sharing and caring, starting with yourself. Love yourself, and by default, you will pass that love on to others, putting you firmly on the road to hair happiness.

Learning checklist

- Make the right entrance. Be the best version of you. The authentic you, not who you think others feel you should be.

- We are all prone to making judgements, which means we all face being judged. Therefore, being true to ourselves is the best way of ensuring the most positive outcome from any interaction we have.

- Just because we all judge – and our brains have evolved to do this to conserve energy – it doesn't mean we should.
- Know that you are likely being judged and how to mitigate it, but become that best version of you, the unlimited you, by learning to reserve judgement.
- Make reserving judgement a habit.

What's next?

You will now be expertly prepared for that next haircut. From understanding the role of your hair in your happiness to the factors you should consider when deciding on your next cut and how best to prepare for this, you couldn't be more ready. You also know how to make the best entrance possible. Now it's time to find out how to make the most of your time in the hairdresser's chair.

9
Keep Talking

Nowhere is communication more important than when you are discussing the details of your cut and colour. Again, ideally you should consult with your hairdresser before your appointment. If not, use the time wisely when you first sit in the chair and the hairdresser asks you what you want today. Talking is paramount to a successful cut and colour, and hair happiness, as is making sure your hairdresser sees your full profile, which we'll come to later.

Ask questions and be curious. Ask for their recommendations. Ask them why they are recommending a particular style. Ask them if they have a lookbook you can go through together. If you've brought one of your own, show it to them.

If they are not forthcoming, initiate the discussion by talking about what you like/don't like about your hair, how you style it and so forth. Essentially, your hair backstory if you've decided to create one. Otherwise, mention what you do for a living and what you like to do outside work. What hairstyles can they recommend? If you dye your hair, ask them if you are getting the colour right for your skin tone, eye colour and life stage.

Typical questions

A great hairdresser will typically ask many or all of the following questions, or versions of them:

- What are you expecting from this visit today?
- Do you know what face shape you have? Would you like me to analyse your face shape and body shape?
- How much time do you have today?
- Do you do anything professionally or in your leisure time that could impact what hairstyle could work best for you?
- How much time do you typically spend on your hair? Is the amount of time you spend dictated by desire or necessity?
- How do you style your hair at home? What styling equipment do you have at home?

How good would you rate yourself at styling your hair? Would you like some tips from me?

- Do you like styling your hair? If not, would you like me to give you some tips on how to make it easier?
- How often do you wash your hair? How do you go about washing your hair? How do you go about styling it from wet?
- If you only wash your hair two to three times a week, what do you do on the days you don't wash it? Would you like me to give you some tips on dry styling?
- What do you love about your hair?
- What do you dislike about your hair?
- What do you want to achieve with your look? What's important to you?
- What have been your best and worst haircuts?
- How brave are you feeling? How adventurous are you feeling?
- If you could have any style in the world, what would you love? (Note: The hairdresser may not recommend the style if your hair type, face or body shape doesn't suit. By asking this question, they are attempting to get to know a bit more about you and what you are thinking.)

The questions are intentionally open-ended to encourage you to talk; the more information you can give the hairdresser, the better. The steps we recommended in Chapter 7 will help you answer the questions.

Struggling to decide what you want in a haircut? Why not think about what you *don't* want.

Each of us can make a difference to the world around us. Here's your chance. If your hairdresser isn't asking many questions, help them learn and grow by sharing what you know. They may just be having an off day and will appreciate you taking the initiative.

A great hairdresser will always be open to learning – or a helping hand – even from their clients. Besides, rapport works both ways and the stronger a relationship you build with your hairdresser, the better for your hair. They will feel more comfortable asking you questions, and you will feel more comfortable opening up. When you communicate effectively, you experience the power of mutual satisfaction or wonderment. That which is good for both can and will last.

The full picture

Having walked through the salon door with purpose and in complete control of any judgements your brain might be trying to make on the quiet, your next task is to ensure your hairdresser sees your full profile. Not the receptionist, not the person handing you the gown, not the trainee washing your hair, but the person styling your hair. Do this before you get too settled in that chair. Ask them if they wouldn't mind looking at you standing up and to recommend styles that flatter your body shape.

This is where a pre-appointment consultation, or holding the consultation away from the styling station, is beneficial, as it will give your hairdresser a chance to see your full profile without the gown.

As the following story about a young journalist, whom we'll call Alice, shows, you fail to do so at your peril.

Alice's story

Alice, a young journalist from a small town, had been handed an exciting assignment by her editor. She was to pose as a customer at a local salon and interview an up-and-coming hairdressing star, whom we'll call John. Alice's editor had heard that John was working for one week a month in a famous London salon and, thanks to one of his hairstyles featuring on the cover of a top magazine, was fast becoming a celebrity hairdresser.

The day of the assignment dawned. Enthusiastic about what was in store, Alice arrived at the salon early, where she was greeted by the receptionist with the news that John was running a little behind but that an assistant would wash and prepare her hair in the meantime.

Returning Alice to the stylist's chair, the assistant asked, 'A coffee, tea or water?' before adding, 'John won't be long. He knows you are here.' Opting for water, Alice settled in the chair to wait.

HAIR HAPPINESS

The water arrived at the same time as John. 'Hi, what can I do for you today?' he asked.

The assignment brief at the forefront of her mind, Alice replied, 'I hear you are becoming quite the hairdressing star. What would you personally recommend?'

John stood behind the chair and looked at her in the mirror. He could see she had an attractive face and that her head was petite. After a few moments of deliberation, he declared, 'Something strikingly different.'

Alice had naturally wavy, shiny dark-brown hair that hung past her waist. Her hair was blessed with strength and vitality, and she loved it. To her, it was a special gift. She desperately wanted to reply 'No, thank you', but she was here to do a job. Swallowing her courage, she told John, 'You're the expert. Do what you think is best for me.'

'May we take a photo at the end?' John asked.

'Yes,' replied Alice, her confidence returning, and she thought, *Maybe I'll make the front page.*

The next hour was like a three-hour horror movie as Alice witnessed an unravelling disaster over which she had little control.

John beamed as he presented the finished cut, but Alice could barely contain the tears. With his phone camera at the ready, John whipped the salon gown away with the flourish of a Spanish matador wielding his cape before *el toro*.

John set great store in his precision-cutting skills, creating a perfect Joan of Arc crop to emphasise Alice's stunning face, but as she stood up, no longer wearing the salon gown, her height and body shape revealed a complete hair design tragedy. Alice was 1.5 metres tall and weighed 70 kilos.

'My head looked like a cupcake on the back of a pig. Utterly ridiculous,' she would later recount.

How long will it take for Alice to grow back 76 centimetres of hair? Healthy hair grows around half an inch a month, so more than two years. How long will it take for Alice to forgive her editor for the assignment? Our bodies and brains remember every pain we experience. How long will Alice blame herself for not saying 'No, thank you'?

Yes, hair grows back, but the trauma of a horrific haircut can remain with us. After all, hair is the gown or suit we cannot take off, so it needs to be treated with the utmost respect.

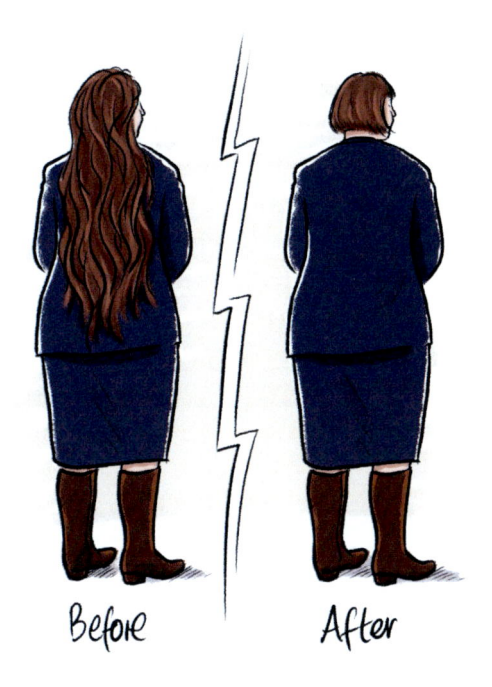

Before   *After*

Alice

Top hairdressers fall into different categories: those who prefer to focus on honing their skills rather than pleasing their clients; those who aim to please and make every effort only for the clients they see as walking, talking advertisements for furthering their careers; and those who see their job as complete the moment the client walks out of the salon.

Thankfully, there is another group of hairdressers: the ones who see it as their life's work to make people happy every single day. Not only on the day of the salon visit but each day in between. These are truly special hairdressers.

If the hairdresser doesn't attempt to look at your full profile, make a point of standing up, moving aside your gown if necessary and asking if the style they are recommending suits your body shape as well as your face shape. Advances in AI should make this process a whole lot easier.

Whatever happens, don't be Alice… or John.

Learning checklist

- Communication is important, full stop, but especially so when discussing your cut and colour. Get this wrong, like Alice did, and you'll be walking around with the consequences for a long time to come.

- There are several questions a great hairdresser will ask you. If yours isn't asking you these questions, and you want to give them the benefit of the doubt, prompt them by raising the questions instead, or prepare and share a hair backstory.
- Make sure the stylist sees your full body profile.

What's next?

Now you are clear on why you are having a haircut, what to expect and the steps we recommend you take before and at the start of your appointment, we will focus on what comes after and how you can make sure you are equipped with the knowledge and tools to ensure you can maintain your hair happiness between cuts.

10
Do It Yourself

If you follow the guidance in the previous chapter, we are confident you will be happy with your haircut. While your hairdresser is working on your hair, or even at the consultation stage, make sure you ask how to manage your fabulous new hairstyle at home. They'll be able to show you how as they style it for you. Being able to easily maintain the style yourself is at the heart of hair happiness.

If your hairdresser conducted a proper consultation at the beginning, you should have a hairstyle that suits your lifestyle and stage, making it easy to manage. The key here is to walk away from the salon with a hairstyle you can effortlessly maintain, leaving you looking fantastic every single day between cuts.

We encourage hairdressers to offer an open-door policy, allowing you to pop in and have a tweak if you are struggling to manage your style, or perhaps a fringe trim between appointments. If your hairdresser isn't forthcoming, ask. Ideally, this should be a value-added service that will build your trust in them and your confidence in managing your new hairstyle. This is where bringing a hair coach onto your team might help, if offering an open-door policy isn't viable for your hairdresser or coming in to the salon between cuts isn't practical (although hair coaches aren't hairdressers, so their support won't go beyond styling advice).

If, after everything, you aren't satisfied, say something. Ask the hairdresser to run through why they recommended that particular cut and style. Be curious. It might grow on you once you understand the rationale (pun intended!). If relevant, ask if they can make some adjustments.

We always recommend you book your next appointment before you leave. Life gets busy, and before you know it three months or more have passed and your hair happiness is on the wane. Hair grows at different rates, as we have shared. Also, some haircuts grow out faster than others. Consult with your hairdresser on the best approach. You may feel you are already well informed and more than proficient in styling your hair, but we guarantee you will still learn something.

DO IT YOURSELF

Life cycle of a haircut

Like so many things, your haircut has a life cycle: the initial cut, growth and maintenance and then the next cut, as illustrated in the diagram below.

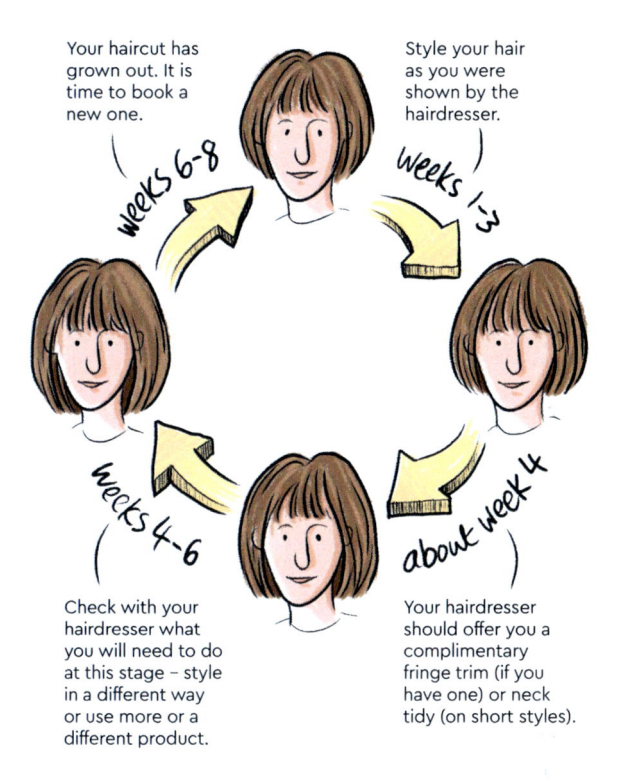

Weeks 6-8 — Your haircut has grown out. It is time to book a new one.

Weeks 1-3 — Style your hair as you were shown by the hairdresser.

About week 4 — Your hairdresser should offer you a complimentary fringe trim (if you have one) or neck tidy (on short styles).

Weeks 4-6 — Check with your hairdresser what you will need to do at this stage – style in a different way or use more or a different product.

Haircut life cycle (for illustrative purposes only – everyone's hair grows at different rates)

This is a general guide. The length of time between appointments will vary depending on your hair type and style.

173

If your hairdresser doesn't offer the information, ask how your haircut will behave in the first two, middle two and final two weeks, working on the assumption you will be going back in six weeks for your next cut. Of course, adjust accordingly based on how long you have agreed with your hairdresser to wait between cuts; the length of time you should wait will depend on the style and your hair type.

Find out how to best manage your hair at the various stages. Will you need to change the brush size and products part way through? Ask them for tips on styling your hair from your perspective – facing your reflection in the mirror – which will be the opposite of theirs. How do you best handle the hairdryer, brushes or other tools while holding them behind your head or across your face?

At the pre-appointment consultation, ask them if it's OK to bring along your own hairstyling kit from home so they can show you the best way to use it. Ask about how often you should shampoo your hair. What type of shampoo and conditioner should you use? How does your hairdresser rate the overall health of your hair and scalp? What should you be doing to keep it healthy or improve its health?

> **Insight from Alison Cooney: A minute**
>
> After each haircut, I give clients a minute while I hang up their gowns. I walk away, telling them to play around with their hair to make sure they are absolutely comfortable with it.
>
> When I return to the chair, I ask them if there are any adjustments they would like. This helps reassure them that they have a happy haircut, or it allows them to ask for their hair adjusted to how they really want it before they get up from the chair.
>
> If your hairdresser doesn't offer this, ask if you can have a moment to play around with it, and don't be afraid to speak up if you would like adjustments made.

Product tutorial

To enrich the conversation with your hairdresser, we will give you a rundown on the products most of you use to clean, nourish, protect and style your hair. Whether reinforcing what you already know or teaching you something new, it will help you have a conversation that will put you on the path to hair happiness. If ever you're not sure, ask your hairdresser for their advice.

Our collective knowledge could easily fill an entire encyclopaedia, so we are sharing what we believe will help kick-start an informed discussion with your hairdresser.

Shampoo

It may sound obvious, but the role of shampoo is to clean your hair and scalp; in particular, removing dirt and excess oil from around your hair follicles. For this reason, we recommended in Chapter 6 that you give your scalp a good massage when you wash it – not only to strengthen the follicles but also to clean around them.

Your shampoo needs to be gentle. Shampooing your hair, especially with warm water, will open the cuticles, which allows the hair to absorb any good nutrients from the shampoo but can leave the hair vulnerable to harm if the cuticles are left open, which is why you should always follow with a conditioner.

If your shampoo was as harsh as, for instance, soap, it would strip away the outer layers of your hair, which we know are essential for protecting the hair's cortex and, therefore, its strength.

The ingredients will give you a clue to how gentle it is. Although this is getting easier, as fewer contain them these days, aim to avoid shampoos with sulphates and parabens, which can potentially strip the hair of its natural oils. As a rule of thumb, the gentler it is, the better it is for you and the environment. The exact shampoo you use will depend on whether your hair is dry, neutral or oily. There are specialist shampoos that help improve volume, reduce dandruff, increase moisture, protect colour and remove excess oil.

Regardless, the one thing that marks out a good shampoo above anything else is its capacity to stimulate growth by keeping your hair follicles healthy, infusing them with vitamins, minerals, nutrients and natural extracts.

Conditioner

As with shampoo, check the ingredients of your conditioner to determine how gentle it is. The role of conditioner is two-fold: it locks moisture into your hair while protecting it from the sun and other environmental damage. You should always use conditioner in tandem with shampoo. Shampooing your hair opens the cuticles to let the goodness in, and conditioning closes them to keep it there. Like shampoo, the type of conditioner you use depends on the nature of your hair.

Serum

This has a number of roles depending on its formulation, from reducing frizz and preventing heat damage to bringing out the shine in otherwise dull hair. Other benefits of using serum include reducing knots and tangles and enhancing your hair's appearance. Serums often contain natural ingredients that nourish the hair – typically argan oil, jojoba oil, aloe vera, coconut oil and the like – infusing moisture into each strand, making it look and feel silkier and glossier.

Serums can include silicone, and it's this ingredient that creates a protective film around the cuticle, reducing the incidence of split ends and frizz. Serum must be applied sparingly and not on the roots.

Mousse

Meaning 'foam' in French, mousse adds volume and makes your hair look and feel shinier. You can use it to give hold and definition, tame curls and make them even bouncier. It can also help reduce frizz. As with products like serum, less is more.

Hairspray

This hairstyling staple has two jobs: to hold your hairstyle in place and add volume. It works by using polymers that bond individual hair strands together so they stay in place. Hairspray can be aerosol or non-aerosol. Both have their pros and cons. Aerosol sprays allow you to apply the hairspray evenly over a wider area but contain less water and more alcohol, which is less beneficial for your hair. Non-aerosol sprays with their pump-action nozzle are great if you need a targeted application, but you would find it harder to get even coverage over a large area. Containing more water and less alcohol, they are healthier for your hair, you and the environment.

DO IT YOURSELF

Gel, waxes and pomades

These are your go-to products when you want your style to stay in place no matter what. Gels are versatile and can help create a variety of styles, from curly looks to messy looks, slicked-back hair, defined partings, topknots and so on. The downside is that your hair can look noticeably stiff, making it obvious you're using a product. Waxes are great on thicker hair and can give your hair shine. Pomades give you the best of both worlds. A combination of a strong hold while looking natural has made them popular among people with thicker hair; they don't work so well on fine hair. Removing the product from your hair, however, can take several washes.

Insight from Sharon Dale: Four rights

I always make a point of talking through the products and techniques I'm using when styling a client's hair.

We call them the 'four rights': the right product for the style, the right amount of product, the right placement (where on the hair) and the right way to apply it.

Otherwise, what can happen is the hairdresser can be busy chatting to the client, applying the product on autopilot, and before you know it, the client walks out with no idea what products to use on their hair and how.

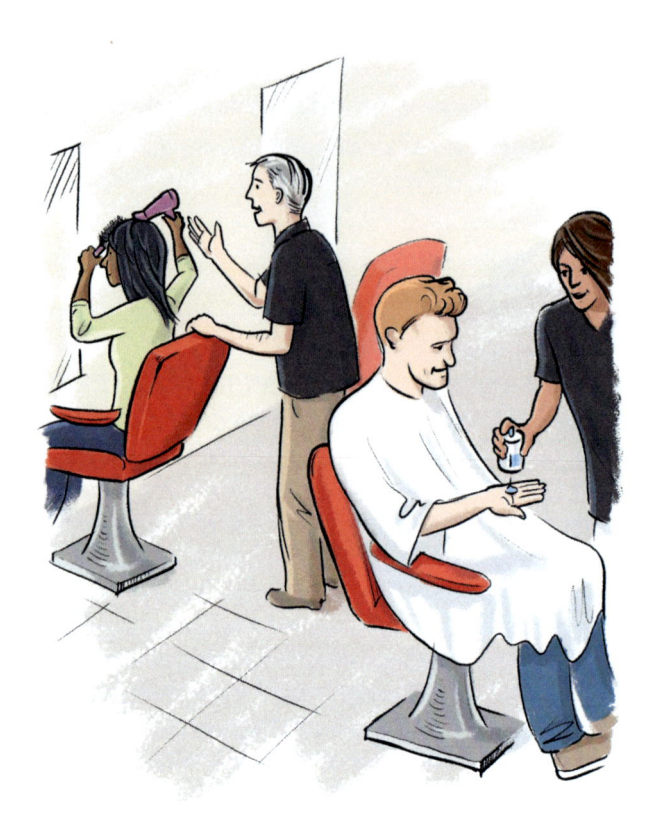

Demonstrating tools and products

Tool tutorial

As with the products, we want to build your knowledge of the styling tools you frequently use or could be using. Again, our goal is to reinforce what you already know and maybe even teach you something new to enrich any discussions you have with your hairdresser.

It is important to remember that when using tools that require heat, *never* apply them without products that protect against heat. There are numerous heat protection sprays on the market, although the products featured above will include varying levels of built-in heat protection.

Hairdryer

The hairdryer you pick should depend on your hair type.

Fine hair: As this is more fragile, ensure whichever hairdryer you choose has a low heat setting. Due to the nature of fine hair, its cuticles are less robust and, therefore, more prone to heat damage.

Other hair types: Choose a hairdryer with a range of heat settings. If your hair is prone to frizz, make sure it has a cold-air button. Blasting your hair with cold air after hot closes the cuticles, giving hair its shine.

Using your hairdryer

Like everything, a good blow-dry starts with great preparation, and that preparation starts in the shower and proceeds through the following steps:

- Wash your hair with *warm* water – not too hot or cold, as temperature extremes can result in brittleness and/or greasiness. The glands that create sebum, the oil found in our hair that, if overproduced, is responsible for making our hair feel greasy, are stimulated by cooler water. Together, the warm water and shampoo will open the cuticles, allowing any nutrients from the shampoo to be absorbed into the hair shaft.

- Apply your carefully chosen shampoo and massage your hair and scalp in circular motions – doing so will improve blood flow to your scalp and stimulate the hair follicles, improving hair growth. It also helps dislodge dry pieces of scalp (yes, dandruff), making it easier to wash away when rinsing. Make sure you rinse the scalp well and the lengths of the hair, too. This will ensure there's no shampoo residue preventing the conditioner from doing its job.

- Using a conditioner you have selected to suit your hair type and needs, work it down the lengths of your hair, focusing on the mid-length to the tips. Don't apply to the scalp this time; it will make the roots of your hair greasy. Leave it for a couple of minutes to be absorbed by the hair before rinsing thoroughly, unless it's leave-in conditioner.

- Gently towel-dry your hair, followed by even more gentle brushing or combing through; when wet, your hair is more fragile and prone to stretching and breakage. For this reason, make sure your hair is about three-quarters dry before reaching for the hairdryer, as drying your hair when wet can damage it. If you are short on time, then rough-dry with the hairdryer. For further protection, apply serum or a heat protection spray.

- It may seem like extra work but investing in clips and sectioning your hair before drying will save time in the long run and result in a better blow-dry. Depending on the length and thickness of your hair, three to four sections should suffice. Start at the nape of your neck, where the most moisture sits, then work up and out. We are aware that not everyone is a fan of drying their hair in the first place. If the thought of blowdrying your hair feels like a chore, but you don't have time to let it dry naturally, a rough dry followed by a once over with tongs, straighteners or another tool recommended by your hairdresser should suffice – not forgetting to apply heat protection first, of course.

- If you want straight hair, dry your hair as you continually brush through. If it's waves you're after, twist and clip sections into loose little buns as you dry. For curls or simple extra volume at the roots, roll your hair around a round brush, and, for better results, increase the heat as you do. Don't forget to give your hair a blast of cold air to reduce frizz and increase shine.

- If you have curly or coily hair, a hairdryer with a comb attachment can help you loosen curls and aid disentangling.

We all have different learning styles, so if it helps you, ask your hairdresser to talk you through this process the next time you are in the salon, or ask your hair coach, if you've decided to bring one on board.

Letting your hair dry naturally

In a world where we are becoming more conscious of our impact on the environment, we thought it only fitting to share some tips on drying your hair naturally. The biggest gain is that you reduce your carbon footprint, but it can have many benefits for your hair, depending on its type. If your hair is fine or not so thick, go ahead and give it a break from heat exposure.

For thick hair, proceed with caution as the hair absorbs and holds the moisture from washing for much longer, which can cause the strand to swell, which can lead to damage. We recommend you give the hair a quick blast with the hairdryer so it's damp and not wet, and then leave it to dry. If your hair is prone to frizz or you want to ensure it has some volume, apply a small amount of gel or mousse.

Straighteners

Wide or narrow plates, ceramic or titanium, maximum heat output, curved or sharp edges – there are a number of decisions to be made when selecting straighteners. Again, it comes down to your hair type and how you want to use them.

Fine hair: You can choose narrower plates if you prefer, and curved edges will allow you to use your straighteners as a curling tool. Go for ceramic plates, as they heat the shaft rather than the cuticle, which is gentler on the hair. They will take longer to heat up and require more passes, but they will be much kinder on your delicate hair.

Thick hair: Wider plates may be the better option, as they allow you to gather more hair in one go and straighten it with fewer passes. Opting for curved edges means greater versatility, as you can use your straightener to create curls. If you have thicker, coarser hair, going for titanium plates is more likely to result in hair happiness – and less tired arms. Titanium plates heat up faster and heat the cuticle, meaning the hair straightens more easily, which is what you want with thicker, coarser, stubborn hair.

Tongs

Like straighteners, it comes down to your hair type when choosing the material and heat settings of your curling tongs, with hair length influencing the size you buy.

Fine hair: Ceramic tongs are best for this hair type; they heat evenly, lessening the chance of heat damage.

Thick hair: Tourmaline tongs are popular with this hair type; they reduce dryness, brittleness and dullness by smoothing the hair cuticles. Titanium is another option; it's lightweight and durable but has a higher price tag. The size of the barrel will depend on the length of your hair. Smaller barrels are good for shorter hairstyles, producing a tighter curl that also makes them great for creating volume, so they are a good choice if your hair is fine as well as short. Medium barrels work well on medium-length hair, and larger barrels that produce waves and big loose curls are ideal for longer tresses.

Brushes

There are so many different types of brush you can choose from, but we will focus on the main brush or brushes you should choose for your hair type.

Fine/thinning/ageing hair: Boar bristle brushes are made from 100% natural soft bristles and are gentle on the hair and scalp, making them the ideal choice for people with fine, thinning or ageing hair. Boars shed their bristles, so come to no harm. The brushes are a by-product of an entirely natural process. Although soft, the bristles are stiff, allowing them to detangle without pulling out the hair. They also redistribute healthy oils across your scalp as you brush, improving the health of your hair and leaving it smooth and shiny. Teasing brushes are an option if you have fine or limp hair. A teasing brush is a small brush employed to tease hair up from the crown to give the impression of fuller hair. They can be a blessing for people experiencing hair loss.

Thick hair: A paddle brush is essential for thick hair, as it allows you to quickly cover a large area while smoothing the hair and giving it shine. Choose nylon bristles if you want a brush tough enough to run through thick hair quickly but go for softer boar bristles if keeping your scalp and hair healthy is a greater priority.

Straight hair: As with thick hair, paddle brushes are well suited to straight hair because you can brush through lots of your hair at once. If your hair is prone to static, a brush with a rubber pad is a good bet, as it has a neutral charge and doesn't generate static energy, unlike plastic. What's more, it allows the bristles to move, so it is softer on your scalp, unlike wood. If you want volume, waves or your hair to curl under, go for a round brush, too. Your hairdresser can advise which size best suits your hair and the styles you want to achieve.

Curly and coily hair: A 'wet hair' brush or a wide-tooth comb is recommended for these types of hair, as is brushing or combing when the hair is still wet.

Wet hair is more elastic and prone to breakage, and both the 'wet hair' brush and wide-tooth comb are designed to be gentle on hair when wet.

Long hair: Again, paddle brushes are a good fit as they allow you to brush large areas of hair in one go, making them effective for brushing long hair. If your hair isn't naturally wavy or full of volume, choose a round brush. You can use a teasing brush to create volume at the scalp for fine hair. We also recommend a good quality boar bristle and nylon combined brush which will detangle without harming long hair.

Short hair: Combs, as a rule, are great for short hair. They are perfect for creating precision partings, as well as for generating volume and feathering or fluffing up shorter styles.

Clippers and trimmers

Clippers have greater versatility. Trimmers are best for precision work. Which type you choose will depend on your hair type and need.

Fine hair: If you have fine hair, you have the option of choosing clippers with magnetic motors, which are low maintenance and affordable.

Thick hair: The main thing to consider is the motor type. Opt for one with a rotary or pivot motor. If you cut when dry, choose a rotary motor, as it has the added advantage of durability – it won't overheat, even when used for long periods. Go for clippers with a pivot motor if you prefer to cut your hair when wet, as the blades will move in both directions, resulting in a speedier cut. You'll also need to bear in mind your choice of blade: stainless steel, carbon or titanium. While carbon and titanium blades help you hold an edge when clipping, carbon blades are prone to rust, and titanium can be costly but is more durable. Stainless steel isn't prone to rust but doesn't produce such a clean cut.

Colouring your hair

Cost savings and convenience make it tempting to dye your hair at home. We get it. Even so, we will argue that it's better to have your hair dyed in the salon, but why? In short, you get what you pay for. Let's look at some of the reasons why.

In a salon, we can professionally advise on the right colour and the correct tone and depth that will not only bring out the best in your hair but also complement your skin tone and enhance your facial features and shape. The result is stunning hair that looks as natural as the hair you were born with. We will also ensure you don't skip that all-important patch test. Tempting as it is, we can develop allergies at any time, even to products we have been using for years.

We can create bespoke colour. Box dyes contain a one-size-fits-all developer that may not suit your hair type; in the salon, your hairdresser will select one that does. Likewise, your hairdresser will have a range of colour tones at their disposal, mixing and matching to best suit you. In some cases, they will use more than one to bring out the best in your features – balayage is a great example and one of the most popular means of doing this.

The dye hairdressers use is of a higher quality. It will have fewer or, in some cases, be completely free of chemicals that can cause damage to hair, which can be difficult to reverse. These include:

- **Ammonia:** Not only does it have an off-putting smell, but it can permanently alter the pH level of your hair. Hair in its natural state is too acidic to absorb and lock in hair dye; slightly acidic hair is good, as the acidity allows the hair cuticle to tighten and remain closed – it's why washing your hair with a little vinegar can make it shine. Ammonia triggers a chemical reaction, turning the hair more alkaline, which causes the opposite to happen – the cuticle to open up. While this allows the dye to penetrate the shaft, it leaves the hair dull, dry and brittle. Even if the dye your salon uses contains ammonia, the hairdresser will be trained through technique and the use of products to limit its damage.

- **Sulphates:** These may strip natural oil from your hair.

- **Hydrogen peroxide:** Found in permanent and semi-permanent dyes, this is the activator that stops the colour in the dye from washing out. While acidic, it works in tandem with chemicals such as ammonia. The latter triggers the hair cuticle to open up, as described above, allowing the hydrogen peroxide to penetrate the shaft and the good stuff to leach out.

There are other chemicals that are found in hair dyes, but your hairdresser will be trained to minimise any risk they pose; for example, by running the mandatory patch testing we recommended above. These are:

- **Parabens:** Preservatives that can trigger an allergic reaction to dyes

- **p-Phenylenediamine (PPD):** The chemical found in permanent dyes and the potential allergen; the darker the colour, the more PPD

Having your hair dyed in a salon will mean you get even coverage, whereas you will struggle when you are colouring your hair at home and relying on your reflection in the mirror along with inadequate lighting. You may not even realise the resulting colour is uneven.

Lastly, we will use high-quality hair products such as conditioners, serums and hair masks that counteract the damage caused by the dye, reducing the alkalinity of the hair and smoothing down the cuticles, which has a dual benefit of locking the colour in and stopping any goodness in the hair from leaching out.

The cost of correcting poorly coloured hair is typically up to double the cost of getting your hair professionally coloured in the first place. As Sarah's story in Chapter 1 demonstrates, the ramifications can go far beyond the cost.

> **Insight from Alison Cooney: Knowing what suits**
>
> A client once asked for vibrant red hair.
>
> 'Orange-red or blue-red?' I asked. 'I don't know which is which,' said the client.
>
> 'Orange-red would suit your complexion better,' I told them, pulling out my lookbook and scrolling to examples of both colours.
>
> 'That one, you mean?' said the client, pointing at the blue-red. 'I love that one.'
>
> But what we like the look of on other people won't necessarily suit us.

It is up to you at the end of the day. Now, at least, your decision will be better informed.

DO IT YOURSELF

Hair extensions

Also known as 'added hair' or 'weaves', these can be used for several reasons, including extending the length of your style, adding a new dimension to your style, such as a different texture or colour, or adding volume. When caring for this type of hair, talk to your hairdresser, but in general, make sure you use the products as recommended by your hairdresser, avoid going to sleep with wet extensions, brush with care and use heat-styling tools with caution.

Bringing it all together

By incorporating the suggestions in this book into your haircare process, you will achieve a positive outcome for both you and the hairdresser, as the following case study shows.

Hair happiness all round

Anya, a mum in her forties, had listened to us talk about many of the topics covered in this book. The topic of the relationship between the hairdresser and the client especially resonated, so the next time she visited the hairdresser, she decided to put what she'd heard us say into practice.

Her hairdresser that day happened to be the salon's creative director. Usually circumspect, Anya was more curious, asking the hairdresser questions about how and why her hair behaves in certain ways. The hairdresser responded enthusiastically, pleased to have someone taking a real interest and revelling in the chance to share her passion.

What Anya learned from the hairdresser was hardly rocket science, but oh, how she could have avoided so much frustration with her hair over the years had she asked before.

Usually relatively prescriptive in terms of the hairstyle she wants, this time, Anya put her trust in the hairdresser, asking her for advice. Of course, she made sure the hairdresser saw her standing and asked what style would suit her body shape. With wide hips, the answer was volume. The hairdresser complimented Anya on her cheekbones – this hadn't happened ever, and Anya was overjoyed. The hairdresser went on to suggest layering to highlight Anya's cheekbones while pulling out her lookbook and showing Anya what styles suited her face shape and why. She also explained that a lighter hair colour would suit her as she aged. Having cut Anya's hair, the hairdresser showed her how to style it at home. 'That was so enjoyable,' said the hairdresser afterwards, 'it hardly felt like work,' and she proceeded to charge Anya at the junior stylist rate as a token of her thanks. Anya loved her new hair, loved the experience. She also loved seeing the hairdresser take so much joy from the process.

DO IT YOURSELF

As covered in Chapter 4, you may not be as satisfied as you'd like with your hairdresser even after taking all the steps we've recommended. That being the case, think about how you can turn the disappointment into something positive. What have you learned? What could you do differently next time? Focus on this rather than on who's to blame. Will you find a better way to work with your current hairdresser, or will you look for a new one?

Learning checklist

- Choosing your cut and colour should extend to how you manage it, if you want true hair happiness.

- Before you even stand up from the chair, make sure your hairdresser shows you how to style your hair. Our product and tool tutorial will clue you up, so you can have a more informed conversation.

- Ask your hairdresser what to expect from your hair as it grows – your hairstyle's life cycle. Find out how you should adapt your haircare routine at each stage.

- Even if you continue to colour your hair at home, you'll be doing so knowing the drawbacks and why we recommend the professional touch.

What's next?

Now you are clear on why you are having a haircut, what to expect and the steps we recommend you take before, during and after, we will delve deeper into the different types of hairdresser, salon and service in our quest to help you become better informed so you can achieve hair happiness.

11
Simply The Best

No hairdresser sets out to deliver a bad haircut, but it occasionally happens and is typically the result of poor communication. Communication is fundamental to hair happiness, as we have reiterated throughout this book. Your hairdresser might even deliver a technically perfect haircut, as John did for Alice, but if it isn't what you want, or it doesn't suit you, then it's of no consequence. Preparation plays an important role, too, which is why the pre-appointment consultation we covered in the last chapter is worth its weight in gold, both for you and your hairdresser.

Still, communication and preparation are only parts of the puzzle. Another critical piece is the chemistry between you and your hairdresser. Your hairdresser might have all the good intent in the world, but their pre-appointment consultation with you is only as good as your ability to communicate with one another, which, in turn, is only as good as the connection you've made, which is, in other words, the oil you need to keep the cogs of your communication turning.

Ultimately, for any of this to work, it's essential you team up with a great hairdresser, one that's right for you. What should you be looking for in your search for the exceptional? How do you find that special someone who will give you a twinkle in your eye? There are no hard and fast rules; at the end of the day, what might be right for you may not be for somebody else.

Before we forge ahead, it's not only your hairdresser who should strive to be exceptional in the pursuit of hair happiness, as you will now be well aware. In many cases, the guidance we share can apply to you, too.

What makes a great hairdresser?

There is no denying that perception plays a role. It comes back to chemistry. Who you perceive to be a great hairdresser and who you get on with will not necessarily be the same for the next person. We will all want different things from a salon. Our opinions on what constitutes a great haircut or service will vary significantly based on our experiences, values, beliefs and current needs.

If we purchased cars without paying any heed to what we wanted in a vehicle – ignoring our values and beliefs – and focused instead on what we felt we needed in a purely functional sense, we'd all be driving the cheapest option that met our criteria.

Furthermore, what we look for in a hairdresser and salon is never constant; it will vary depending on what is going on in our lives. Take dining, for example. Sometimes, all we are after is to quickly fill up with fast food, while at other times, nothing less than fine dining will satisfy us. The same can apply to our hair.

Having said that, there will always be a standard below which few of us will be prepared to go – one where what are known as 'hygiene factors' have at least been met.

Hygiene involves more than soap and water

Hygiene factors are the basics you should expect from every hairdresser or salon – the absolute minimum requirements. If a hairdresser doesn't meet them, you should avoid them at all costs. They include a safe salon environment, a clean hairdressing station, a trained hairdresser, a hairdresser you can communicate with – that is, you speak a mutual language to a competent level – a comfortable seat, warm water for washing your hair, a clean gown and clean towels.

From bad to great, different hairdressers might approach these factors in the following ways:

- A **bad hairdresser or salon** will offer less than the hygiene factors. Shocking, but true.

- An **indifferent hairdresser or salon** will offer the hygiene factors, but nothing more.

- A **good hairdresser or salon** will offer more than the hygiene factors, aiming to deliver a level of service that will keep clients coming back. What you consider to be good, though, will vary depending on your own perception.

- A **great hairdresser or salon** will continually seek to go above and beyond. They will take genuine pleasure in delighting their clients and will do everything in their power to ensure that every client continues to experience that feeling each and every day between cuts. They see themselves as purveyors of joy not only to their clients, but also to the wider community.

Vidal Sassoon summed it up perfectly: 'Hairdressers are a wonderful breed. You work one-on-one with another human being and the object is to make them feel better and to look at themselves with a twinkle in their eye.'[11]

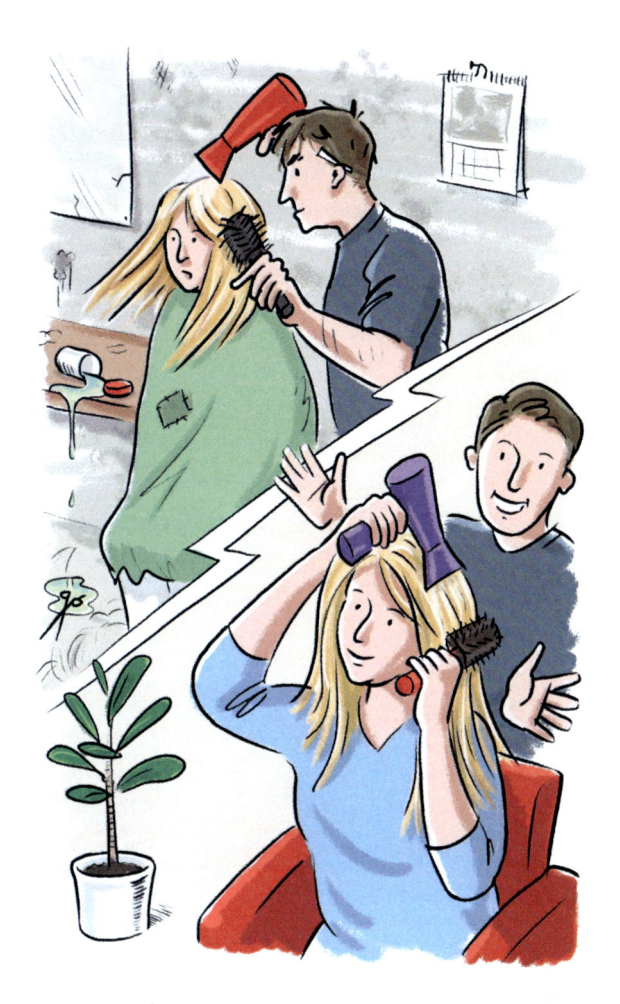

Bad vs great

They see hairdressing as more than a job

Is it clear your hairdresser loves what they do? Do they inject passion, energy and enthusiasm into whatever is asked of them? Are they continually striving to be the best they can? Are they a purveyor of joy? Are they proud of who they are and what they do? At 365 Day Hairdressing, we turned work into play and played to win. If your hairdresser loves what they do and strives for excellence, that can only benefit you.

Do they see hairdressing as a vocation, or do they view it as a means to earn money? Ideally, it should be both. While we want you to find a hairdresser who sees their work as more than a job, we encourage hairdressers not to shy away from aspiring to earn more. If your hairdresser believes in themselves and their potential and they have a strong sense of self-worth, you will benefit.

There is nothing wrong with any of us loving what we do and earning plenty at the same time. It comes down to having a positive money mindset – one where we don't allow limiting beliefs to trap us in a negative relationship with money, our capacity to earn and our self-worth. It is something all of us should keep an eye on so we don't shy away from wanting to earn more while doing something we love.

They surprise, delight and entertain you

Anyone driven by passion will have an intrinsic desire to surprise and delight. Has your hairdresser ever done more than you expected or even thought possible, such as tuning into your mood and talking you out of a potential hair disaster? For instance, twigging that the complete restyle you are asking for is driven by a recent breakup, and while it might make you feel better for five minutes, you'll regret it later.

Exceptional hairdressers are great at reading people. As we shared in Chapter 4, the uncanny ability to tune into and gauge your mood and emotional state and adapt their approach accordingly while interpreting a whole range of nonverbal signals that you don't even realise you are giving off is one of their superpowers.

One of 365 Day Hairdressing's co-founders, the wonderful Stephen Way, asserted that having your hair cut should be an experience. He would insist that his stylists learn a different skill – including magic, juggling or singing – simply to entertain their clients.

They are consistent and understand you

Being exceptional doesn't happen by chance. It takes effort and commitment. Continuous success isn't an accident; it is by design, and consistency plays a big role. Put simply, consistency builds trust and respect, which, in turn, build loyalty.

A great salon or an exceptional self-employed hairdresser will have set up processes and systems to ensure their clients always experience the best service. This doesn't mean a one-size-fits-all approach – the opposite, in fact. The client will consistently receive the service they expect, but a bespoke one that has been crafted to them: a perfect balance of consistency and individuality.

Accordingly, 'the best service' will look different to each of us, centring on what we value as important – taking time or being efficient, for example, or a friendly, talkative stylist versus one who is quieter. We each have different personalities, values, likes and dislikes. Does your hairdresser understand yours? Is the chemistry there?

On the subject of talking, are they curious? You may want a quieter stylist, but you also want one who takes time to find out about you and what you want.

They regularly go the extra mile

How much effort do they make to establish what you are looking for? Do they offer the chance to discuss your hair wants and needs before the appointment? As we said at the start, preparation is paramount. To help you apply this to your hairdresser, consider the following questions:

- Do they ask questions about your lifestyle and current health? These are both relevant to your hair.
- Do they look beyond your hair? Have they ever advised on face shape – and glasses if you wear them – and how your hair fits into the mix?

Have they offered you advice on your make-up? Would you feel comfortable asking them?

- Do they ask you to stand up so they can properly assess your profile, face and body, or do they consider it beyond their remit? If the latter is true, it's a shortsighted folly on their part, as the former will always result in much better outcomes, with the return considerably higher than any additional effort invested – remember Alice!

- Do they help you to become a DIY hairdresser? Are they generous with their time, advice and guidance, or do they closely guard their skills and experience, afraid to relinquish any authority or power, not realising that they are achieving the exact opposite?

- Do they show you how to style your hair at home and offer advice on products and styling tools? Do they suggest you bring them to the appointment so they can give you their opinion, or are they set on recommending only the products and tools favoured by the salon? Again, this is a shortsighted approach.

- Do they offer open-door maintenance? A lesser salon or hairdresser will shy away, mistakenly writing it off as loss-making. A great salon or exceptional hairdresser will welcome it with open arms. Wise. We know it encourages loyalty.

They share loyalty, trust and respect with you

Loyalty is built on trust. Do you value and trust your hairdresser's advice? Do you respect them? Do you feel they respect you and value your custom? They might demonstrate this in the following ways:

- They are open with you and admit when they don't know the answer. Perhaps they go and seek advice from a colleague rather than trying to answer your question themself, and they are not afraid to seek counsel from others in their team so they can give you the best possible advice.

- They treat one another with respect, If they don't, what does that say about how they treat you, their client? They might be polite to your face, but what about once you have walked out of the salon? If they don't treat people with kindness and respect as a rule, can you trust that they always give you the best advice when it comes to your hair?

Any hairdresser worth their salt will know that what we do not value, we do not protect, and what we do not protect, we lose. They will, therefore, be keenly aware that, in addition to being a good person, it's in their interests to make you feel valued and, as a result, win your trust, loyalty and respect.

Having said that, while it will be important to them that you value their advice, they won't want you to completely defer to them.

They work with you, not on you

Have you ever been an Alice and instructed your hairdresser to do what they want with your hair? Did they push back? What questions did they ask? Did they constructively challenge you? Did you end up with a better haircut and style as a result, or did they take everything at face value and just do what you asked without questioning? What was the outcome? If it did work out, you got lucky.

True, an exceptional hairdresser wants you to value their advice, but they understand that hair happiness can only be achieved with your input and that they don't have a carte blanche to do whatever they want with your hair. When they ask you to contribute, they are not copping out. They know that looking after your hair is, and should be, a team effort.

In our increasingly busy and faster-paced lives, it's tempting to treat our salon visit as a chance to kick back, relax and let someone else take over. Change your mindset. You need to play an active role in having your hair cut. Go prepared, be present, make suggestions and ask questions. An exceptional hairdresser will expect this from you.

If your hairdresser is willing to take over completely while you switch off, treat it as a red flag. Remember John. Remember Alice.

They are open to trying new ideas and approaches

Perhaps you have come across a new style or approach while researching your next cut. A good measure of how open your hairdresser is to working with rather than on you is their willingness to learn and to give the idea a try. Are they curious? Do they ask questions to find out more, or do they strike the idea down cold when it's barely out of your mouth?

Attitude is important, as is a willingness to learn and improve, as we have said before. It reflects the spirit of the true artist and professional, for an overdone strength will quickly become a weakness.

Everything needs a healthy balance. Anyone who believes they have honed their craft and don't need to continue learning – from those more experienced *and* from those less so – will soon fall behind.

It's worth remembering that what's not growing is dying. You should be looking for a hairdresser or salon committed to maintaining state-of-the-art standards of knowledge, skills and techniques to enhance their personal and professional performance. One where it is obvious every member of the team, from the newest apprentice up, is empowered to suggest ideas and take the initiative, fostering an environment of continuous growth and improvement.

Regarding the new kid on the block – the hair coach – does your hairdresser view them as a threat or an opportunity to provide you with an even better service?

If you use a salon rather than a self-employed hairdresser, and your current salon is a place where only the salon management's word goes, and it is one where you can see unnecessary crises or self-imposed deadlines created or manufactured, then it's time to move on.

A collaborative approach

If you are a salon user, do you feel you are being looked after by the team as a whole? Do you sense a camaraderie among the hairdressers? Is it fostered by the salon management? Going back to our earlier point about trust and respect, how do the hairdressers in your salon treat one another? Are they quick to help each other out and share advice to make sure you get the best service? Have you observed the hairdressers learning from one another? Naturally, you want the team to be strong, as they will continually learn and improve – to your benefit.

An organisation is judged by the quality of the people it retains. Do you know, or is it obvious, that the salon you use invests in their staff? Hairdressing is a shared endeavour – not only between you and your hairdresser, as we have discussed thus far, but also between your hairdresser and their colleagues, be it in person or online.

If you have answered no to any of the above questions, remember that, while we might not be able to say the same for your hairdresser, although we hope we can, by reading this book and taking on our recommendations, at least *you* will be growing as a person. Depending on your particular circumstances, you can opt to look for a new salon.

Alternatively, you can use your newfound knowledge to build and improve your relationship with your existing hairdresser or salon. In doing so, you will be leveraging your good fortune by sharing it. Think of it as the butterfly effect we touched on earlier. A small act, such as reading this book, or even a single chapter, can result in something much bigger, benefitting you and others.

Taking the first step to learning something new is easier than many of us think, especially when we are supported by others. Sharing is caring, and the world is so much better when we do.

SIMPLY THE BEST

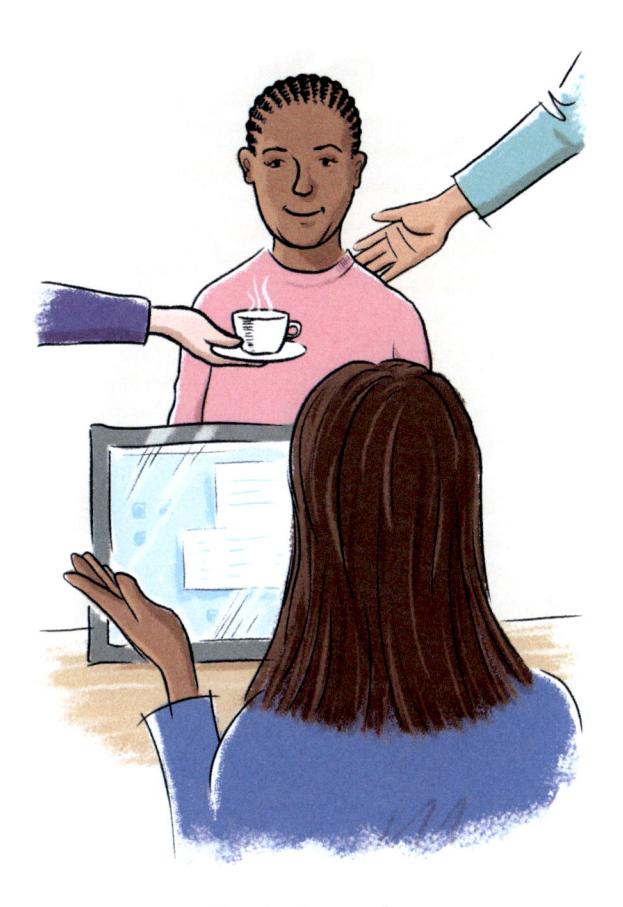

Great salon service

> **Insight from Sharon Dale: Which salon?**
>
> Which salon would you prefer, one where you are greeted warmly by the receptionists and all the hairdressers on duty, or one where you are perfunctorily greeted by the receptionist and ignored

by everyone else while you wait for your hairdresser? A salon where you are offered something to drink and team members who aren't too busy to come and chat with you while you wait if they can see you're open to that, or one where you're sat waiting alone as team members mill around chatting to one another or looking at their phones?

At our salon, we make an effort to make every client feel welcome to the point that our regulars often remark that it feels like walking into a club where they are valued members.

Doing something for the greater good

On the subject of sharing, you can tell the measure of a business by how it interacts with the community it belongs to. Does the salon give off a vibe of each for themselves and take, take, take? Are staff driven mainly by what's in it for them, or do they believe they have a responsibility to those around them, be it caring for the environment or helping those in need? If you use the services of a self-employed hairdresser, what impression do they give you?

The basis for doing good is not purely altruistic, although that may be what motivates us on a conscious level. It actually does *us* good to help others; our brains release nature's mood boosters – oxytocin, serotonin and dopamine – when we do.

As an added bonus, these mood boosters counteract the effect of cortisol, which is triggered when we are under stress. Hairdressing, as a service profession dealing with something so crucial to a person's identity and happiness as their hair, can be stressful at times. A hairdresser, or salon and team, that proactively helps others will be healthy in mind, body and spirit, which will positively impact their professional skills. Once again, this benefits you.

Great value for money

After all is said and done, do you feel your visits to the hairdresser are great value for money? We don't mean a cheap haircut. We mean an optimal return on your investment. You want your hair to feel like the gift that keeps on giving.

Shift your mindset

As you will now know, hair happiness results from many things, including your attitude and behaviour. Like in any area of life, you are drawn to certain types of people as they are to you. The client–hairdresser relationship is no different.

If your hairdresser suggests a different salon or hairdresser, don't be offended. Make the choice not to take it personally. See it as them having your best interests at heart – whatever their motivations. If it's a great salon, their motivations will be honourable. On the flip side, even if you love your hairdresser, if after reading this book you know deep down that they are not the right hairdresser for you, take courage and move on. Be kind and considerate when you do, but if they take offence, remember it's their choice, just as it would be yours were the boot on the other foot. We are not being unkind when we say this. We simply don't want you to feel responsible for other people's feelings – especially if it's something you're prone to do.

It's down to you and you alone to discover the guiding star of self-worth and discovery that lives within us all – your unlimited self. The unlimited you. We achieve what we believe. If we believe we can have hair happiness, we will achieve it.

> **Insight from Sharon Dale:**
> **The importance of chemistry**
>
> I know that I attract a certain type of clientele, and I don't shy away from it. Chemistry is so important to the client–hairdresser relationship.
>
> Every colleague I have worked with has told me my clients are the most difficult. I disagree with them completely. I love them, and they are great human beings. We work together well.
>
> If you aren't gelling with your hairdresser, find one you do gel with. Don't settle. Your hair is too important.

Insight from Alison Cooney: The art of listening

After each appointment, I take a couple of minutes to note down what we chatted about, even the smallest of details, which I quickly review before the next appointment.

I then make a point of asking them about any specifics they shared at their previous appointment; for instance, the trip to Rome they mentioned they were planning or how their anniversary party went. It makes a great conversation starter. I also note down anything they say they like and dislike, making sure, for example, that they are offered a hot drink with milk alternatives if they have said they're vegan.

They love it and are always impressed, asking me 'How did you remember that?' As hairdressers, we want you to know we value you and are listening.

I make a point of keeping up to date on current affairs. If the client is in a reticent mood and the silences feel awkward, I can, therefore, easily fill them. It also helps build rapport, as it can sometimes reveal a common interest.

I have learned to judge when the client wants peace and quiet and not to try to initiate small talk. It will only irritate them and risk them closing up when I need them to talk.

Reading people and their moods is as important a skill for a hairdresser as any technical skill. It is a key part of communication, and if we misjudge the client's mood, it will only result in a communication breakdown and hair unhappiness, no matter how technically sound the cut.

Learning checklist

- Choose the best hairdresser, but the one that's best for *you*.

- Hairdressers and salons aren't created equal. There are bad, indifferent, good and great hairdressers. You should be aiming for great, but how exactly great looks will be different for each of us. You need to start with looking at yourself and what you want and need; you will have gained a range of knowledge and tools to help you from reading this book.

- There are a number of traits that make a hairdresser and salon exceptional.

- If your current hairdresser isn't measuring up, change them.

What's next?

Now you know how to ensure you are working with the best hairdresser for you and the steps you need to take to achieve this if required, we are going to wrap up by examining the pros and cons of selecting a salon hairdresser over a mobile hairdresser.

12

There's Nowhere Better Than Home – Or Is There?

These days, we are spoilt for choice when choosing where to have our hair cut. Until now, we have spoken mostly about salons and the hairdressers who work in them, but mobile hairdressers or hairdressers working out of a home-based salon or a salon suite (also known as a hairdressing suite) are also an option when deciding to get your hair cut.

Deciding where to get your hair cut

Various factors will influence your choice; how you view them will depend on what matters most to you.

Convenience and price

Convenience may drive your choice to have your hair cut at home. Perhaps you have children whose hair needs to be cut at the same time, or you struggle to find the time to get to the nearest salon, or it's just too far away. Maybe you are living with a health condition or have mobility issues that make having your hair cut at home the preferable option.

Perhaps you get your hair cut at the hairdresser's home salon just down the street, or you may choose to have your hair cut in a salon because it's close to your work and it's easy to pop in during your lunch hour or after work.

Ditto for a hairdressing or salon suite, the hair and beauty industry's version of a co-working space. If you use a freelance hairdresser, they may operate out of a small suite they rent in a space alongside other beauty practitioners. It is a town or city-centre option for freelancers not wishing to operate from a home salon or on a mobile basis that allows you to have your hair cut by your favourite hairdresser in a salon-type setting.

Typically, a mobile hairdresser can charge less, as they have fewer overheads – a contributing factor in favour of having your hair cut at home.

'The one'

You have found 'the one'. You have bonded and work well as a team. They even feel like part of the family.

What's more, reading this book has greatly validated your high opinion of them. Maybe they work in a salon and have no plans to leave. Perhaps they are the owner, or you met them in a salon, and they have decided to go freelance, so you follow them to their rented salon suite studio, or they now come to your home. You fit around them because you simply don't want anyone else working on your hair.

Your personality type

Are you more extrovert than introvert or vice versa? Are you excited by the prospect of walking into a salon, or does it fill you with dread? Yes, we spoke about how to overcome this earlier in the book, but another option is to have your hair cut at home or in a hairdressing suite, where available. Some people love the buzz of a salon, of having their new hairstyle complimented as they leave. They love the opportunity to people-watch. Others prefer the peace and quiet of home or a salon suite.

Flexibility

Working with a freelance hairdresser may give you more scope to suggest new ways of doing things, and vice versa. Not tied by long-held conventions in a salon, they may be quicker to adopt new technologies and new ways of reaching out to you and managing the hair life cycle from virtual pre-appointment consultations to virtual between-cut check-ins, including support with how you style your hair.

The influence of social media

Social media has made it easier to choose a hairdresser, right down to a particular skill set. Are they fantastic at balayage, fauxhawk, keratin treatments and so on? You can see their full portfolio of work within a few clicks. You can have a consultation via instant messaging or chat within moments of reaching out to them, and you both can make a quick decision about whether to work with one another. The growth in hairdressing suites has facilitated this, as it combines the flexibility and directness of freelance hairdressing with the professional equipment available in a studio. Having said that, a growing number of salons won't hire a new hairdresser unless they can demonstrate they have an active and effective social media presence to showcase their work.

Pause for thought...

There are some other factors we'd like you to consider before we part company. They may further reinforce and even heighten the esteem in which you hold your existing hairdresser and choice of venue. Bear with us, though; what we share might give you some valid pause for thought.

As we have said, the guidance we share could indeed validate your past or current choice of hairdresser. Still, if you have fallen into the habit trap, we are confident that our insight, borne out of many decades of experience, will help you make an informed decision about where to have your hair cut going forward.

We'd also like to make it clear at this point that where and how a hairdresser chooses to work has no bearing on their skill and professionalism. It's down to their preferences, more often than not driven by lifestyle choices, just as where and how you get your haircut is down to yours.

Do they keep their skills as sharp as their scissors?

Industries are continually evolving, as are the professional skills required to excel in them, and this is no more true than in hairdressing.

When a hairdresser becomes self-employed, it's on them to keep their skills and expertise up to date. This can work in their favour, as they can have complete autonomy over the areas they specialise in and the nature of the continuing professional development (CPD) they undertake. Hairdressers, of course, are not born equal, and some will be more eager to invest in themselves than others.

Does your hairdresser give the impression that they are keeping up with industry trends? Are they on a self-development track and investing in their own professional skills? The secret to achieving this is being part of a strong team, as we discussed in the last chapter. For self-employed hairdressers, this could mean a virtual team, which we will come to shortly.

The same goes for a salon. How much a salon owner decides to invest in professionally developing their hairdressers will vary, and not all salon-based hairdressers will engage in the training they have been asked to undertake with equal enthusiasm.

Beyond continuing professional development

What about opportunities for informal development? In a well-run salon, it can become part and parcel of working alongside other hairdressers: chatting to colleagues about trends and techniques, picking up tips from more experienced team members or sharing knowledge with those less experienced. If you use a salon, do you see this happening when having your hair cut?

Technology has made it easier for hairdressers working outside of salons to create virtual teams. Do you know if your hairdresser is active in online hairdressing groups? Do they meet up with other hairdressers? Do they team up with others in the industry, not necessarily hairdressers, to improve their expertise and to seek ways to provide you with the best experience and service possible?

THERE'S NOWHERE BETTER THAN HOME – OR IS THERE?

Nothing beats being part of an in-person salon team, but we accept the market is changing, with an increasing number of hairdressers choosing to go it alone, which may breed new life into the industry. Regardless, sharing knowledge, whether face to face or virtually, is essential for any professional. We are not designed to operate entirely alone, and we're not just talking about hairdressers; no one is.

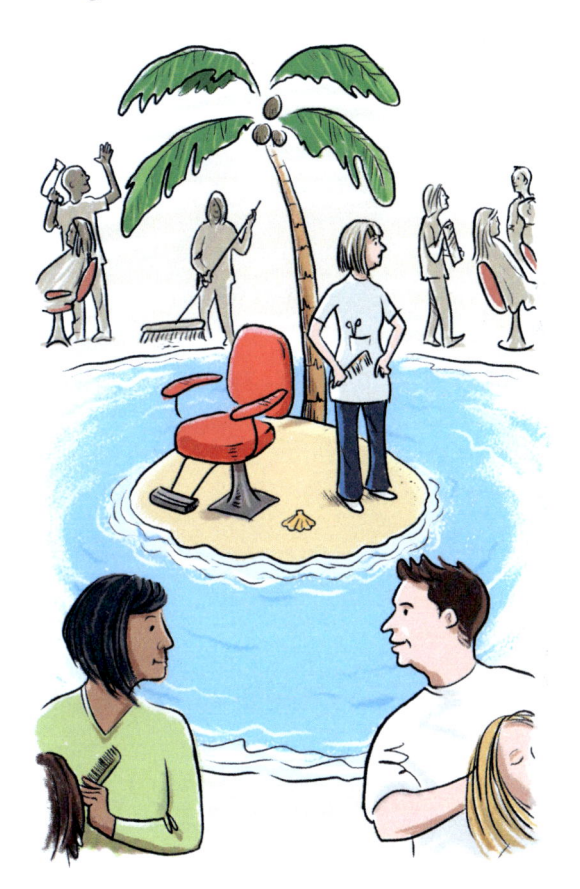

No hairdresser is an island

Consider it a red flag if your hairdresser extolls the virtues of working alone. This is especially true if they are not undertaking any kind of professional development to keep their skills up to date.

Social creatures

Why do we place so much importance on being part of a team? It's not only about sharing tips and techniques. We humans are social creatures, and, while there will always be exceptions, most of us find that we are the best version of ourselves when we can interact with others regularly. We thrive on it, even.

There is growing evidence that we need social interaction in the same way as food, water and shelter – so much so that a substantial part of our brain is given over to encouraging it. In fact, being deprived of social interaction for long periods can cause changes in our brains. That's how fundamental it is.

We are not saying that hairdressers opting to work independently are depriving themselves of social interaction – of course not. They will regularly interact with you and their other clients. It is also highly unlikely that they behave like hermits elsewhere in their lives.

Our point is that we are the best version of ourselves when we work in a team. For our ancestors, belonging to a community became essential for survival, as being alone left them vulnerable to predators. Over time, our brains have evolved to thrive when we interact with others and actively seek to belong, particularly with those similar to us.

While going solo may benefit your hairdresser in terms of flexibility and autonomy, they should nevertheless find time to interact with other hairdressers if they want to be the best they can be. The same goes for hairdressers working in a salon. If the hairdressers in your salon don't appear to be interacting as a team, treat it as another potential red flag.

Why other hairdressers and not just anyone? All types of social interaction are essential, whether in person or online, with people similar to us or those who stretch our socialising abilities, but it is especially so with people who share our interests and with whom we can find a common language – for instance, those who have chosen the same career.

In addition to making us feel happy and fulfilled, surrounding ourselves with like-minded and supportive people changes how we respond to stress. Evidence shows that our blood pressure and heart rate remain lower if we have supportive people at our sides when facing challenging situations.

As we have explained before, hairdressing can be stressful. For the sake of your own hair happiness, you want the best for your hairdresser, which means a hairdresser who is well supported – whether remotely or in person; ideally, both. With so many specialist groups on social media, it's never been easier for them to find their people.

Of course, coming out and asking them would feel intrusive, and it is not what we are suggesting you do. Having reached this point in the book, however, you will have a good measure of the type of person your hairdresser is, whether they are a solo traveller or value sharing and learning from others and giving and receiving support.

Perils of too little variety

As the saying goes, there are two sides to every coin. We clearly benefit from surrounding ourselves with the familiar and with people from whom we can draw comfort. Still, we need variety and a willingness to proactively embrace the unknown if we want to excel. Like we have said before, an excess of something is never good.

As a rule, a hairdresser working in a salon cannot pick and choose their clients. This has its advantages in that it helps them maintain their skills, keeping them sharp; they never know who will turn up in their chair beyond their regulars.

A self-employed hairdresser, on the other hand, has complete autonomy over the clients they work with, which is clearly a benefit for the hairdresser, but what about you, the client? When a hairdresser cuts the hair of only a select few regulars, their skills will naturally lose their edge where they have fallen into the habit of cutting the same hair in the same styles.

If a hairdresser is not exposed to observing colleagues trying new techniques or working with a variety of clients requiring them to use different skills, their skill set can become narrow and dulled. As we liked to remind those who went through the 365 Day Hairdressing programme, that which is not used is lost. This includes your hairdresser's skills. Meanwhile, as their client, you could be missing out on new trends, not to mention a style that may suit you better than your current one.

What can hairdressers do about this?

If you happen to be a hairdresser reading this and our words have hit home, what can you do to keep your skills fresh and sharp? If you're self-employed, perhaps you could work one day a week or a couple of days a month in a salon, or hire a chair within a salon?

Form or join collectives with other self-employed hairdressers renting studios nearby or working out of their homes or on a mobile basis to share tips and knowledge and support one another? Look for hairdressers online with similar interests. Unlike generations of hairdressers before you, the world really is your oyster, and you could be sharing or taking advice from fellow hairdressers across the globe.

Learning checklist

- There are many factors influencing whether you choose to entrust your hair to a salon or a self-employed hairdresser and there are pros and cons to each option – for you and the hairdresser.
- Factors such as variety, CPD and skills maintenance should be considered. How well does your hairdresser fare on these?
- As ever, there is always something you can do about it.

What's next?

We still have a bit more to share, but we are moving away from your hair and heading into the realms of what cannot be seen: the gut. Ultimately, paying this often-undervalued part of you some overdue attention will help you achieve hair happiness for a long time to come. Intrigued? Keep reading.

13
Gut instinct

Tragically, in November 2023, Leslie was diagnosed with pancreatic cancer. Despite bravely facing his illness head-on with the mix of curiosity, determination and positivity that was so typical of him, he sadly passed away in May 2024. One thing Leslie's diagnosis taught him was that many of us, himself included, take this vital part of our bodies for granted. The irony wasn't lost on him – having taken a closer look in his final months of life – that the role of the digestive system in our happiness is more considerable than many of us imagine. Here are his thoughts on the subject:

> 'Part way through writing this book, I was given the news none of us want to hear: "You have cancer." In my case, pancreatic. Once

the initial shock of the diagnosis subsided, I began to question how much attention I had really paid to how I had fed and nurtured my body over the years. As a lifelong learner, I already knew a considerable amount about the workings of the digestive system and its role beyond breaking down and facilitating the absorption of food and other sources of nutrients into our bodies. However, in the context of my diagnosis, revisiting the subject really brought home the incredibly important role of the digestive system in our happiness. I am not talking about the tangible happiness you feel on eating your favourite meal, but the role of the gut in our nervous and endocrine systems and their impact on our emotional and physical well-being and, ultimately, our happiness.'

The second brain

We spoke briefly in Chapter 6 about the impact of nutrition on the health of our hair, how it improves the appearance and texture from within and how that impacts our happiness, along with everything else we have covered in this book. Hair happiness is, however, more than skin-deep. Here, we will lead you away from the surface – and what we can see – and take you into the inner depths of our digestive system – or into the bowels, you might say.

Our gut, essentially our digestive tract, is increasingly referred to as the second brain, and rightly so. For instance, 95% of serotonin, the neurotransmitter responsible, among other things, for making us feel happy is created in our gut. It is also argued that more than 50% of dopamine, also responsible for happiness, but more in terms of reward and motivation, is generated there.[12,13]

How much serotonin and dopamine we produce is directly related to the volume of good bacteria we house in our gut's microbiome. Regularly eating foods that inhibit the production of good bacteria will reduce the amount of serotonin and dopamine our gut generates, which, in turn, will lower our mood. It will also impact our sleep: melatonin, a hormone that regulates sleep, is made from serotonin, so the amount of melatonin we produce is proportionate to the amount of serotonin available in our gut. Less serotonin, less melatonin, greater sleep disruption.

If we sleep less, we will have less energy, impacting our mood further. Our energy levels will also be affected by the nutrients we absorb, which are the direct result of what we eat, as well as how effectively our gut absorbs them. This can, in part, be related to our diet, its impact on our gut's microbiome and the volume of good bacteria our gut contains; specifically, how well these good guys break down our food and facilitate absorption.

Gut health can also be due to underlying health conditions or genetics. If you have a health condition that affects how well your gut absorbs nutrients, you may have been advised to change your diet or, where necessary, embark on a programme of gut healing using pre- and probiotics or similar.

Either way, taking care of your gut is integral to your overall health and well-being, whether you can optimise it by making simple adjustments to what you eat or need extra support. If you have not treated yours as well as you might, do not despair. You have not consigned yourself to a life of misery.

We are what we eat, but all is not lost

While studies have suggested that our microbiome is well and truly established by our third birthday,[14,15] we can still make changes to the health of our gut throughout our lives, which will lead to positive outcomes that reach far beyond our digestion. As such, the eating and other lifestyle habits we foster and their influence on our microbiome and the healthy functioning of our gut will directly impact our happiness. We are what we eat, and we are in control of that.

In short, a healthier gut results in greater happiness. It really is as simple as that, and everyone has it in them to make positive changes to their diet that will result in a happier life.

If you are struggling to find the motivation, consider this: how you feel about yourself can impact the health of your gut and other areas of your body. Even if the first step is a challenge, healing your gut will help you heal your mind, which will, in turn, result in greater gut health and an even stronger mind.

Mind-body connection

We have established that there is a strong connection between our mind and body. This connection isn't, however, limited to the gut. When we experience a traumatic event, large or small, our body remembers it. Although emotional in nature, over time, the impact of the trauma can affect our health physically, manifesting in our body as pain, high blood pressure, migraines and gastrointestinal problems, to name just a few. What happens in our lives on an emotional level will impact us on a physical one – good and bad.

What's more, we may think we have a handle on whatever life throws at us, perhaps putting the odd aches, pains and other niggles along with changes to our skin and hair down to growing old or a need to slow down. Our mind, however, subconsciously processes many of our emotional experiences, triggering the chemical responses to those emotions, including stress, without us knowing. This, in turn, triggers reactions in our body, so it is worth considering whether there is more to those aches and pains.

Coming full circle, as we have already hinted, you can become more resilient to stress through better gut health; higher serotonin and dopamine levels mean lower cortisol levels, as hindering the production of this stress hormone is another thing they are known for.

Make the change from the inside out

As you can see, what we eat and drink can influence how we feel, and, as we have learned, how we feel can impact our appearance. It can work the other way, too – feeling good about how you look can make you want to take better care of yourself in other ways. Go with whatever works best for you.

Going from the inside out, however, will lead to more sustainable results, as a healthier body and mind will help you establish the habit of looking good. As they say, beauty comes from within. During his illness, Leslie shared these thoughts:

> 'I can honestly say I have lived my life to the fullest with few regrets, but if there is one

thing I could change, it would be to take much more care of my digestive system.

'It goes without saying that I have achieved hair happiness, along with happiness in other aspects of my life. But could my path to hair happiness and, indeed, overall happiness, have been easier with better gut health? And how does this relate to my pancreas?

'Yes, it could have been, not least because my mind and body would have been inherently better at handling stress. Furthermore, would it have meant I could have used mindfulness, meditation and the many other techniques I have mastered over the years to better effect?

'My pancreas, in turn, would have had an easier time of it. The rich food and alcohol we like to consume, often in the pursuit of happiness, will have made it work overtime.

'I am not suggesting you cut out such food and alcohol completely; just be mindful of what you are asking your body to do each time you partake and the true impact – short- and long-term – that it has on your happiness. As I have said throughout this book, an excess of anything is never good.'

If you are fortunate not to have an underlying condition affecting your ability to absorb nutrients (and plenty of tests are available these days to check this), you can take control of your gut health and happiness by being more mindful about what you eat.

Talk to a professional

If Leslie's story and the guidance he shared have prompted you to examine your gut health, please seek out one of the many amazing nutritionists, nutritional therapists or other gut health specialists there are. They can advise on any necessary investigations, dietary adjustments or other methods of gut healing.

There you go – the final piece of the puzzle when it comes to your happiness, hair and everything else: your gut.

Learning checklist

- Hair happiness is more than skin deep.
- What goes on in our gut can impact the health of our hair – as well as our overall health.
- The gut is often referred to as our second brain. An impressive 95% of serotonin, the neurotransmitter responsible for happiness, among other things, is made in our gut. In healing our gut, we can heal our mind.
- We are what we eat, but all is not lost if our eating habits leave much to be desired. We can improve our gut health at any stage in our lives.
- Our emotional state can impact our digestion (and many other areas of our health) so it's worth

being mindful of whether there is more behind those aches and pains than a dodgy takeaway or a pulled muscle.

- If any of this resonates or causes concern, please talk to a professional.

Conclusion

There we have it. Perhaps you have been putting our advice into action as you go along, or perhaps you have decided to read the book before taking any action. Whichever applies to you, you should be well on your way to hair happiness or thoroughly prepared to embark on the journey. As you may have gathered, happiness is a journey, not a destination. You can start achieving happiness today; it's not something you have to wait for.

Flick back through the book and pick something that comes to you easily. It will help you take that crucial first step. Like all things worth working towards, achieving happiness with your hair and in your life will take effort. Some steps might feel like they come naturally, but others will challenge your current beliefs and drive you to change your behaviour, your mindset and how you approach your relationships with yourself and others. They will take practice and perhaps leave you doubting yourself. Which ones they are will depend on you, your hair, your life experiences, your relationship with yourself and your hairdresser.

There will be times when you think, 'Why didn't I start doing this years ago? It's so obvious!' Be kind to yourself – we only know what we know at the time.

We'd love for this to be a journey you take with your hairdresser. Now that you've finished reading the book, why not share what you've learned with them if you haven't already? You could even gift them a copy of the book? Then work with them through the steps that are most relevant to you. Enlist them as your cheerleader. Cheerlead them.

If, after reading this book, you realise you need to change your hairdresser, use what you've learned to find the right one for you. Be discerning – you and your hair deserve it.

If you are a hairdresser reading this, we'd love for you to take what you've learnt and apply it to your clients. Encourage them to read it too.

CONCLUSION

Ultimately, trust in what we've shared with you, and it will take you to a place where:

> 'Every day is a gift of opportunity to laugh, to learn, to achieve, to improve. To make someone happy and to be happy.'
> — Leslie Spears (1937–2024)

Notes

1 R Euba, 'Humans aren't designed to be happy – so stop trying', *The Conversation* (19 July 2019), https://theconversation.com/humans-arent-designed-to-be-happy-so-stop-trying-119262, accessed 23 April 2025
2 MG Efran, 'The effect of physical appearance on the judgment of guilt, interpersonal attraction, and severity of recommended punishment in a simulated jury task', *Journal of Research in Personality*, 8/1 (1974), pp45–54, www.sciencedirect.com/science/article/abs/pii/0092656674900440, accessed 24 April 2025
3 W Kirsch and W Kunde, 'On the origin of the Ebbinghaus illusion: The role of figural extent and spatial frequency of stimuli', *Vision Research*,

188 (2021), pp193–201, www.sciencedirect.com/science/article/pii/S0042698921001711#b0065, accessed 24 April 2025

4 L Buscaglia, *Love: What life is all about* (Ballantine Books, 1996)

5 V Richardson, 'Men more ruffled by bad hair', *The Guardian* (27 January 2000), www.theguardian.com/uk/2000/jan/27/1, accessed 24 April 2025; see also E MacBride, 'Researchers: A few bad hair days can change your life', *Insights by Stanford Business* (11 April 2014), www.gsb.stanford.edu/insights/researchers-few-bad-hair-days-can-change-your-life, accessed 24 April 2025

6 The University of Texas Permian Basin, 'How much of communication is nonverbal?' (no date), https://online.utpb.edu/about-us/articles/communication/how-much-of-communication-is-nonverbal, accessed 13 February 2025

7 T Schwartz, 'Six keys to changing almost anything', *Harvard Business Review* (2011), https://hbr.org/2011/01/six-keys-to-changing-almost-an, accessed 13 February 2025

8 C Handy, *The Age of Paradox* (Harvard Business Review Press, 1995)

9 T Schwartz, 'Six keys to changing almost anything', Harvard Business Review (2011), https://hbr.org/2011/01/six-keys-to-changing-almost-an, accessed 13 February 2025

NOTES

10 A Rice, 'Trauma-informed mindfulness: A guide', *PsychCentral* (5 January 2022), https://psychcentral.com/health/trauma-informed-mindfulness, accessed 24 April 2025

11 hjadmin, 'Vidal Sassoon's 12 most inspirational quotes', *HJ Magazine* (17 January 2017), https://hji.co.uk/vidal-sassoons-12-most-inspirational-quotes, accessed 24 April 2024

12 N Terry and K Gross Margolis, 'Serotonergic mechanisms regulating the GI tract: Experimental evidence and therapeutic relevance', *Gastrointestinal Pharmacology* (2016), https://link.springer.com/chapter/10.1007/164_2016_103, accessed 18 February 2025

13 Y Chen, J Xu and Y Chen, 'Regulation of neurotransmitters by the gut microbiota and effects on cognition in neurological disorders', *Nutrients*, Jun 19 (2021), 13(6):2099, doi: 10.3390/nu13062099

14 RE Moore and SD Townsend, 'Temporal development of the infant gut microbiome', *Open Biology*, 9/9 (2019), https://royalsocietypublishing.org/doi/10.1098/rsob.190128, accessed 24 April 2025

15 M Derrien, A-S Alvarez, WM de Vos, 'The gut microbiota in the first decade of life', Trends in Microbiology, 27/12 (2019), pp997–1010, www.sciencedirect.com/science/article/pii/S0966842X19302148, accessed 24 April 2025

Acknowledgements

In my grandfather's final days, he spoke about this book with such fondness. He made it clear that whatever the future held for him, he wanted the book to be completed. I was honoured to pick up the mantle and, working with the fabulous team he had brought on board, ensure Leslie's wish to see this book published was granted and in the most fitting way possible.

Thank you to Tanya Gaffon, who spent many an hour talking with Leslie about the book and whose conversations and tireless effort to keep the book going while Leslie focused on his cancer treatment were a source of joy and solace for him in his final months.

A special thank you to Keith Chandler for being a wonderful friend and incredible business partner to Leslie for more than five decades, for agreeing to contribute his priceless knowledge and expertise to the book and for setting aside time to work with Tanya to complete the book in the months following my dear grandfather's and his dear friend's sad passing.

An equally special thank you goes to Sharon Dale and Alison Cooney for their unwavering friendship and unstinting support of Leslie's vision for the hair industry and for contributing their invaluable technical knowledge and expertise, as well as a wealth of insider knowledge that has unquestionably helped to bring this book to life.

Thank you to Keith's partner, Tory Hart, and everyone else who gave up their time to review the book and provide their input. Finally, thank you to the team at Rethink Press – Sarah Marchant, Anke Ueberberg, Kathleen Steeden and Tess Jolly – to Jez Duncan for his beautiful illustrations, and to the tens of thousands of hairdressers and salon professionals who passed through 365 Day Hairdressing and our salons, without whom we wouldn't have been able to craft and hone the expertise shared in this book.

George Spears

ACKNOWLEDGEMENTS

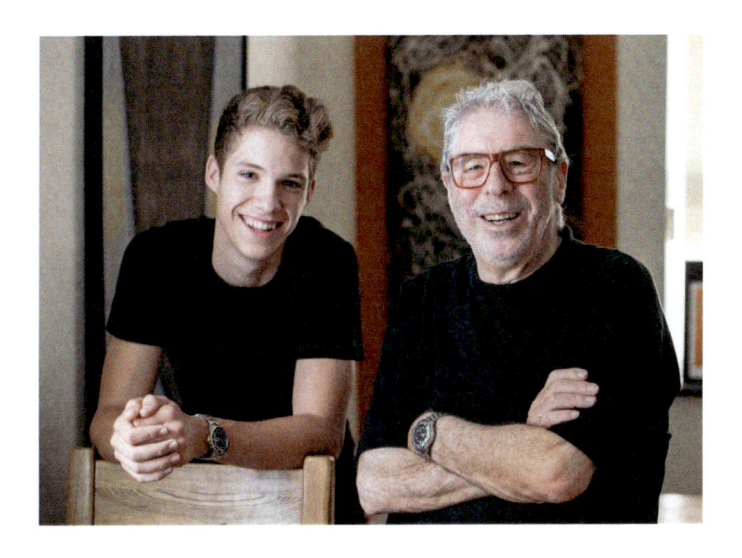

George Spears and Leslie Spears

The Authors

Leslie Spears

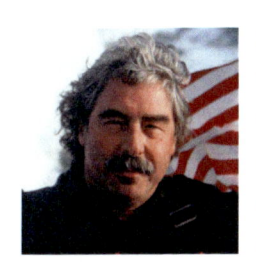

Born in London in 1937 into a world on the cusp of war, Leslie went on to live a remarkable life, shaped but not defined by the circumstances in which he lived his earliest years.

Leslie's experiences as a child during the war and directly after – separation from his family, long-term illness and its impact on his education – forged him into the man he became, endowing him with the grit and determination to overcome his disadvantaged start along with the steadfast compassion and desire to promote joy in his life and those around him.

His professional success speaks volumes – of a person committed to making the most of the years granted to him and leaving a positive mark on the world, from teaching himself to read in his twenties, a move which allowed him to propel himself from the shop floor to behind a desk and then further into the ranks of managing and leading global companies, to ultimately creating, building and leading his own – 365 Day Hairdressing – transforming an industry and the lives of many as he went. These efforts were justly crowned when he was jointly recognised alongside Vidal Sassoon by the Fellowship of British Hairdressing in 2000 for his outstanding contribution to the hair industry.

365 Day Hairdressing transformed how hairdressers perceive hairdressing and its role, and theirs, in our lives. The concepts that Leslie, and others in the 365 Day Hairdressing family shared tirelessly, instilled in a generation of hairdressers and salon owners a conviction that our hair and those who help us care for it play a role far more significant than they had previously been given credit for. Joy Ltd continues this work, building on the importance of cultivating joy, for those working not only in the hairdressing industry but also far beyond.

Coming from a man who was the epitome of kindness and generosity and who gave so much throughout his life, it is fitting that this book is Leslie's final gift to the world.

THE AUTHORS

Keith Chandler

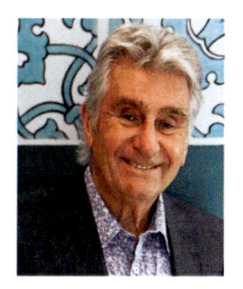

Now a resident of the Sunshine State, Keith was born and raised in England.

Having passed the eleven-plus, Keith received a traditional English grammar school education, but, unlike many of his peers, he opted out of attending university. Instead, he chose to continue his learning in the workplace, securing an engineering apprenticeship within the UK automotive industry and following it with a degree in mechanical engineering.

Taking this less conventional route served him well. Within a few short years of working for the UK's largest motor distribution group, he rose to become its youngest-ever regional director, running fifteen UK dealerships in addition to the company's French subsidiaries in Bordeaux and Toulouse.

It was during this period that Keith first met Leslie Spears, but it wouldn't be until a decade later that their destinies would merge, changing not only their futures but also an entire industry and the lives of many in it for the better.

Meanwhile, continuing his upward trajectory, Keith relocated to Southeast Asia, where, for the next five years, he oversaw two multinational trading groups as chief executive.

Returning to the UK in 1982 and concluding that he wanted to build businesses rather than run them for others, Keith launched the first of what would become a chain of auto dealerships. The venture proved successful, growing to seven locations and US$50 million in sales.

With his reputation as an accomplished business leader now firmly established, it was not long before Keith was invited to deliver management courses for the prestigious Dale Carnegie Institute in the USA.

Yet change was on the horizon in the form of an event in 1984 that would alter the course of his career forever and herald the start of a love affair with the hair and beauty industry that endures today.

Aware of Keith's training credentials, now long-time friend Leslie Spears invited him to share his management expertise with pioneer members of Leslie's newly launched 365 programme. It sparked an epiphany in Keith, who realised that while hair was as far as you could get from cars, he was where he was meant to be.

Keith and Leslie's partnership grew and strengthened to the point where, in 1991, Keith joined Leslie's latest venture, Salon Success, eventually becoming Global Director of Education, and where, over the next three decades, he developed and delivered industry-redefining salon education programmes in the UK, Europe, the USA and Australia.

Today, Keith divides his time between running Joy USA, his distribution company based in Tampa, Florida, where he now resides, and as chairperson of Joy Ltd, a role he took on following his dear friend Leslie's passing.

His passion for education, nevertheless, remains unabated, and he is keen to share his ideas and principles with an ever-wider audience.

Keith believes that it is his obligation and that of other leaders of today to pass on their given talents and skills to the leaders of tomorrow. Surrounding himself with a select group of outstanding people who always drive him to be the best version of himself, he has shared his management philosophies in no fewer than thirty-two countries.

His approach to life is simple: 'Treat each day as the beginning of the next, and best, ten years of your life.' This mantra has certainly held true during his forty-year love affair with the hairdressing industry.

Sharon Dale

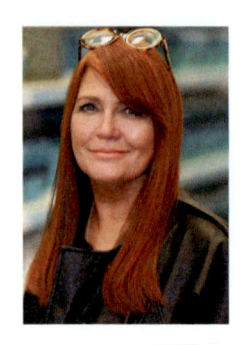

Born and raised in South London in the 1970s, Sharon drew on an innate mix of grace, grit and determination to overcome barriers many would find insurmountable and fulfil her dream of becoming a top hairdresser – qualities that continue to serve her well.

A talented hairdresser with a career spanning more than forty years, Sharon developed and honed her craft under the watchful eye of the late Stephen Way after walking into his West End salon at the tender age of fifteen and pitching for a job.

Spotting something special, Stephen hired Sharon there and then, and when Leslie came knocking in the mid-1980s in search of someone to test his new 365 concept, Stephen knew she was exactly what Leslie was looking for. Sharon stepped up to the challenge, and the rest, they say, is history.

Sharon spent many years accompanying Stephen and Leslie all over the world, sharing her now sought-after hair styling expertise at leading industry shows and training and changing the lives of countless hairdressers.

After stepping back to get married and have children, Sharon returned to work with Leslie in the mid-2000s, joining the Joy Ltd family, where she remains and is determined to continue Leslie's legacy.

Alongside, and as a testament to her much-deserved status as a top hairdresser, Sharon has spent several years fronting up designers at London Fashion Week as well as acting as lead hairstylist in association with Moroccanoil at the Eurovision Song Contest.

Alison Cooney

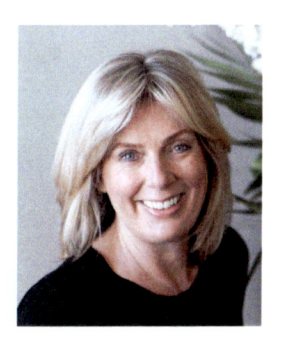

Fresh out of school and just sixteen years old, Alison began her hairdressing journey in 1984 in Taunton, Somerset, where her passion for the industry developed over the next five years. Then, in 1989, she ventured to London to work in not one but two career-defining roles: with renowned stylist Stephen Way in his esteemed New Bond Street salon and as a lecturer and in-salon educator with celebrated industry disruptor Leslie Spears at 365 Hairdressing.

When still in Taunton, Alison had participated in a series of 365 Day Hairdressing Business Builder courses, where she attended lectures by Stephen and

Leslie. Inspired by their expertise and the 365 concept, she took the decision to work with them in London.

It marked a significant shift for Alison, who had previously lived on a remote West Country farm.

During her five years in London, Alison honed her skills while gaining invaluable styling experience in the theatre, television and radio. She also became a lecturer alongside Stephen and Leslie for the same 365 Day Hairdressing Business Builder courses she had attended in the West Country, enriching her knowledge and network.

In 1995, she returned to the West Country to start a family, though she continued her collaboration with Leslie at Salon Success, focusing on client service and hairdressing standards.

Just under a decade later, in 2004, Alison co-founded The Mount Salon with her business partner and sister. Their combined expertise in hairdressing, business and customer care led to rapid success, and the salon remains a thriving business.

Driven by a desire to always learn more, in 2009, she partnered with Leslie to introduce the Moroccanoil brand to the haircare market as a distributor. Now a freelance hairdresser for Moroccanoil, Alison has been privileged to participate in prestigious events like

THE AUTHORS

London Fashion Week, influencer product launches, Salon International and the Eurovision Song Contest.

Today, she works three days a week behind the chair at The Mount Salon as a stylist and has just celebrated forty remarkable years in this dynamic industry.